Eat, Drink, & Weigh Less

OTHER BOOKS BY MOLLIE KATZEN

Moosewood Cookbook

The Enchanted Broccoli Forest

Still Life with Menu

Pretend Soup and Other Real Recipes:
A Cookbook for Preschoolers and Up

Mollie Katzen's Vegetable Heaven

Honest Pretzels and 63 Other Amazing Recipes for Cooks Ages 8 and Up

Mollie Katzen's Sunlight Café: Breakfast Served All Day

Salad People and More Real Recipes:
A New Cookbook for Preschoolers and Up

OTHER BOOKS BY WALTER WILLETT, M.D.

Nutritional Epidemiology

Eat, Drink, and Be Healthy:
The Harvard Medical School Guide to Healthy Eating

MOLLIE KATZEN & WALTER WILLETT, M.D.

Eat, Drink, & Weigh Less

A Flexible and Delicious Way to Shrink
Your Waist Without Going Hungry

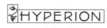
HYPERION

NEW YORK

Printed in the United States of America.

For information address:
Hyperion
77 West 66th Street
New York, New York 10023-6298

Library of Congress Cataloging-in-Publication Data
Katzen, Mollie
    Eat, drink, and weigh less : a flexible and delicious way to shrink your
waist without going hungry / Mollie Katzen, Walter Willett.—1st ed.
       p. cm.
    Includes bibliographical references and index.
    ISBN 1-4013-0249-1
    1. Reducing diets. 2. Weight loss. I. Willett, Walter. II. Title.

RM222.2.K364 2006
641.5'635—dc22

          2005055119

BOOK DESIGN AND TYPESETTING BY:
Pauline Neuwirth, Neuwirth & Associates, Inc.

Hyperion books are available for special promotions and premiums. For details contact Michael Rentas, Assistant Director, Inventory Operations, Hyperion, 77 West 66th Street, 12th floor, New York, New York 10023, or call 212-456-0133.

First Edition
1 3 5 7 9 10 8 6 4 2

CONTENTS

ACKNOWLEDGMENTS

W E ARE HUGELY indebted to Steve Siegelman, whose master skills of prose, understanding, optimism, and passion were key to the birth of this book.

Many thanks, also, to Christine Swett, who assisted greatly and cheerfully with many tasks ranging from recipe tests to research and data organization—and sometimes on very short notice.

David Ludwig, M.D., and Meir Stampfer, M.D., Dr. P.H., were gracious enough to read the manuscript and share their expertise and tremendous knowledge.

We are grateful to our very supportive team at Hyperion, which included Mary Ellen O'Neill, Will Schwalbe, Kelly Notaras, Bob Miller, Ellen Archer, Claire McKean, Ruth Curry, Anne Newgarden, Miriam Wenger, and Ruba Abu-Nimah, as well as the entire marketing and publicity departments. We'd also like to thank Cheryl Forberg, R.D., for her excellent nutritional analyses of the recipes.

Various friends, relatives, and colleagues were available to give feedback and personal testimony that greatly informed our approach to this project. We want to thank Jami Snyder, James DeZutter, Doug Wheeler, Felicia Kruger, Eve Shames, Tresa Smith, Stacey Kaufman, Jennie Kaplan, Duncan Cleary, Sarah Goodin, Robert MacKimmie, and Betty and Leon Katzen for their generous, interesting, and helpful comments.

Walter also thanks his wife, Gail, for support and good meals while working on this project and Debbie Flynn for making sure it moved forward along with other ongoing research activities.

NOTE TO THE READER

THE RECOMMENDATIONS IN this book are not intended to replace or conflict with the advice given to you by your physician or other health professionals. All matters regarding your health require medical supervision. Consult your physician before adopting the suggestions in this book. Following these dietary suggestions may impact the effect of certain types of medication. Any changes in your dosage should be made only in cooperation with your prescribing physician. Before using any vitamins, be sure to consult with the appropriate medical authorities and check the product's label for any warnings or cautions.

Pregnant women are advised that special precautions may pertain to diet. If you are pregnant, talk to your doctor before undertaking any dietary suggestions and before taking any nutritional supplements.

The authors and publisher disclaim any liability directly or indirectly from the use of the material in this book by any person.

Two Roads, One Message:
How and Why We Came to Write This Book

Walter

FOOD, IN ONE way or another, has always been part of my upbringing, my life, and my work. Like many other pioneer families, the Willetts left New England generations ago to find a better life farming the fertile flatlands of the Midwest. My family cleared forests in Michigan to plant crops and graze dairy cows, and did so for nearly 150 years.

Producing food was a major part of my life while growing up. I belonged to 4-H clubs and the National Junior Vegetable Growers Association. At Michigan State University, I studied food science and learned about the use of technology to process, preserve, and distribute food.

Fascinated by the ways in which food affects human health, I decided to go to medical school at the University of Michigan, and then did my internship and residency in internal medicine at the Harvard Medical Service of Boston City Hospital. While this experience was rewarding in many ways, it was also frustrating, because I came to realize that the typical problems of our patients, such as heart disease, diabetes, and cancer, were seldom cured and often unsatisfactorily managed.

Wanting to better understand the root causes and potential prevention of these conditions, I pursued a doctoral degree in epidemiology at Harvard School of Public Health, which gave me a new way to understand the origins of human disease. Back in the late 1970s, nutrition was mainly studied in animals and test tubes, or in small, short-term studies in humans. To understand how dietary factors influence risk of cancer and other diseases, long-term epidemiologic studies in large populations were clearly needed. I decided to make that my life's work.

I began to develop and test standardized questionnaires to assess dietary intake that could be used in such studies. Fortunately, I had begun working on the Nurses' Health Study, which had just been launched by Dr. Frank Speizer to investigate the effects of oral contraceptives on risk of breast cancer, and this population of 121,700 women presented an ideal opportunity to study the long-term effects of diet.

In 1980 we sent our dietary questionnaire to participants, and we have continued to update this information ever since. In 1986 we added 52,000 men via the Health Professionals' Follow-up Study, and in 1989 we added another 116,000 women in the Nurses' Health Study II. These studies have provided a wealth of information on the relation of diet to cardiovascular disease, cancers, and many other conditions that has been published in hundreds of scientific papers.

When we started our studies, many beliefs about diet were not supported by hard evidence, and many aspects of diet that have turned out to be important, such as trans fats and glycemic load, were not even considered by most nutritionists. And we now know that the impacts of dietary choices go far beyond what we were thinking about in 1980. The idea that dietary decisions could impact risk of birth defects, cataracts, and infertility was well outside the mainstream of medicine at that time.

Right from the start, the ultimate goal of our research has been to provide information that can be used to improve health. By the late 1990s we realized that the findings needed to be compiled in a way that would be readable by any interested person. Thus, with the support of Harvard Medical School Publishing and the help of my colleagues, I wrote *Eat, Drink, and Be Healthy: The Harvard Medical School Guide to Healthy Eating*. Because no study should be viewed in isolation, that book is a summary from all sources of the best available evidence on diet and health. Readers of *Eat, Drink, and Weigh Less* who would like more detailed information on diet and health should find it helpful.

As a physician, I have found the response to *Eat, Drink, and Be Healthy* to be highly gratifying. Starting several months after it was published, I was inundated with emails and notes from readers saying how the book had changed their lives for the better. Many motivated people had been led to believe that healthy nutrition meant two things: avoidance of fat and deprivation. From *Eat, Drink, and Be Healthy* they learned how a balance of healthy fats, carbohydrates, and protein sources—along with generous intake of fruits and vegetables—could improve blood cholesterol fractions and glucose levels, and make weight control easier.

Readers were experiencing these benefits and also had an enhanced sense of well-being and control of their lives, which can occur within just weeks or a few months of better eating and regular physical activity. And in many ways, these short-term payoffs are just as important as the prevention of major diseases down the road. I was also gratified that many of my fellow physicians, whose training, like mine, did not include much information about nutrition and who typically do not have sufficient time to discuss diet, found the book to be helpful in guiding their patients.

Although weight control is the topic of a chapter in *Eat, Drink, and Be Healthy*, the continuing increases in overweight and obesity in the United States and worldwide suggested that a book with a focus on weight control could be particularly helpful. In fact, probably fewer than 10 percent of adults living in a modern society where food is abundant and physical activity is unnecessary can successfully control their weight without conscious effort, so this is an issue for almost all of us.

Any strategy for weight control should start with sound nutrition but also needs to address the purchasing and preparation of foods, and how cooking, eating, and exercise fit into the complex lives that we live. For this, additional expertise was needed. Fortunately, I had come to know Mollie Katzen through the Nutrition Roundtable, sponsored by the Department of Nutrition at Harvard School of Public Health. Mollie, through her *Moosewood Cookbook* and other classics that followed, was the culinary guru of my generation who introduced us to new and more nutritious ways of preparing meals. She has championed delicious, healthy eating for more than thirty years.

Mollie's approach to this book has been gentle and flexible, which is essential because almost everyone wanting to control weight lives in a unique set of circumstances, and begins from a different starting point. No one's life is static. And that means that any successful long-term strategy for weight management and healthy eating has to be adaptable to a wide range of circumstances and needs to be varied and enjoyable to be sustainable. Mollie was the ideal collaborator for turning our best knowledge into a usable, real-world plan for everyone.

Mollie

LIKE WALTER, MY lifelong interest in food has consistently taken me beyond the simple needs and pleasures of the everyday table, and into the realm of curiosity and quest. Growing up urban in the era of TV dinners, frozen vegetables, and instant pudding (all of which, I must confess, I loved as a child), I was struck by my first encounter with a vegetable garden at the age of twelve, and spurred by the realization that green beans did not, in fact, grow in the freezer. At that point I dove headfirst into the exciting world of cooking with "real things" procured directly (or recently) from Mother Nature, and I have never looked back.

In my high school years, I spent a good deal of time in the kitchen (thank you, Mom) and began experimenting with recipes using novel (to me, anyway) ingredients like cauliflower, garlic, winter squash, not-from-a-can beans, and mushrooms. Many edible revelations later, in college, I learned about macrobiotic cooking under the tutelage of a Japanese cook in a small café in upstate New York. This was followed by a two-year stint in a very fresh, cutting-edge, "beautiful people" eatery in San Francisco, just when colorful, mostly vegetarian food, inspired by a broad spectrum of joyful ethnic cuisines, was arriving at the margins of American meat-and-potatoes consciousness.

When I took all this experience with me back to upstate New York in the early 1970s to open up a smaller, less flashy version of the same concept, it was well received by the "alternative lifestyle" community and looked upon as something cute and *niche* by the general public. But when this general public relaxed its arm's-length "maybe" attitude and came in to taste the asparagus soufflé that we were selling for $1.50 per (generous) portion (with salad!), many people were won over.

Slowly and steadily, this cooking—an homage to the brilliance of pure agriculture—took root, so to speak. At some point, the hand-lettered recipe journal I'd been keeping this entire time morphed into the *Moosewood Cookbook*, which went on to become a best seller (still out there to this day). But during my period of discovery, when this journal began, I had no idea—not even a premonition or a clue—that this would or could become interesting to the mainstream. All I knew was that I loved cooking fresh from the garden and orchard (or, barring that, from the farmers' market or produce department), and I wanted to learn as much about this world as I could.

And so it happened that during the early and middle years of Walter's research—and well before our acquaintance—I was at parallel play, busily cooking and writing the healthiest recipes my intuition and limited nutritional knowledge could envision. I assumed that vegetables and fruits and a diet centered low on the food chain, was healthier than one centered on meat and processed starch, and I wanted to convert as many people as I could, not to omitting meat from their diet, but to including more of the green growing things.

But even though it turns out I was on the right track in my vegetable enthusiasm, I operated on many of the same assumptions as the general population about what healthy eating might or might not be. I did not yet understand the importance of good fats, for example, and for a while was as embracing as everyone else in America (except, perhaps, Walter and his colleagues) of the low-fat fad and the notion that leaving meat out of a diet automatically conferred greater health, regardless of what was actually consumed.

Somehow, many of us came to define a good diet by the *absence* of things: Say no to meat! Say no to fat! Say no to carbs! I began to wonder where the "yeses" were. How could health be defined by what was *not* consumed? Was it a good thing that many young vegetarians were eating mostly bagels and nachos, and that being a vegetarian often had everything to do with not eating meat and nothing to do with actually eating vegetables? What was a *truly* healthy diet? And, if needed, what would a balanced, sensible, vege-centric weight loss plan look like?

The purpose of my work has never been to convert the world to a meatless lifestyle. I've never wanted to impart a negative message about food. My true passion, rather, has been to spread the Good News about how wonderful healthy eating could be. So I have wanted to reach people with the right, positive message, but I needed to know the science. I was busy with eggplants and apples, brown rice and tofu, almonds and strawberries, and now I also wanted to be busy with learning—and spreading—helpful, sound information.

Fortunately, right at the time of this realization, I also became aware of the research being done by Walter Willett at the Harvard School of Public Health and in the Nurses' Study. It was the early 1990s—a time when the Mediterranean Diet (very strongly connected with and influenced by Walter's work) was making headlines, and lightbulbs began flashing for me and many others.

Several years later, I was honored to receive Walter's invitation to join the new Nutrition Roundtable at the school—a group of people in the food world who would attend meetings to learn about the latest nutrition research being conducted by Walter and his department. For me, it was another epiphany. And it was enlightening, refreshing, and quite thrilling to acquire the tools necessary to put the pieces of the healthy eating puzzle together—to learn about real findings and get beyond assumptions and popular yet unproven notions.

When Walter and I compared notes, we realized that both of us had been asked repeatedly for our vision of a good, logical, and balanced non-fad way to lose weight and keep it off. It soon became clear to us that we would make a complementary team for getting the word out about healthy weight loss and lifelong maintenance, as Walter speaks fluent Science, and I know how to turn his findings into Dinner and then some.

My goal was, and still is, to find the most appealing and delicious ways to prepare and present fruits, vegetables, whole grains, good oils, legumes, and nuts—and dairy, and, yes, meat, if desired—and to get people eating beautifully, and feeling and looking wonderful. I am very fortunate to have found the world's best partner for getting this message out. We hope this book will refresh, enhance, and prolong all of our lives.

Eat,
Drink,
&
Weigh
Less

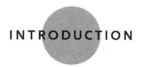
Eat, Drink, and Weigh Less:
A Formula for Weight Loss *and* Better Health

GETTING BACK TO WHAT'S TRUE, REAL, AND GOOD FOR YOU—*AT YOUR OWN PACE*

D IET BOOKS, DIET centers, diet Web sites, diet gurus! They keep proliferating, showing up in different shapes, colors, and sizes. And that just makes it harder to figure out what will work—and work for *you*. So why one more? Well, for exactly that reason. It's time to dial down the noise and get back to the real foundations of healthy weight and lifelong wellness: eating what's good for you, combined with regular exercise. The *Eat, Drink, and Weigh Less* program will show you how.

Our message is not gimmicky or trendy, but then neither is your health. It's important. It deserves truth, not hype. So we set out to strip away all the conflicting information, misinformation, and pseudo-information and went back to bedrock: decades of solid research, fundamental truths about nutrition, and natural foods that have always been our best source of life and health.

Eat, Drink, and Weigh Less is based on the best available evidence from studies conducted around the world, including Walter's thirty years of research about diet and long-term health. It is the result of ongoing, large-scale studies from which many other diets borrow when they need science to support their claims and assumptions. This book will take you right past all the flashy fads and half-truths, straight to what you need to know to achieve and maintain a healthy weight.

Eat, Drink, and Weigh Less is a set of principles, guidelines, menus, recipes, and real-life tools designed to give you just the essential, practical information you need, so that, through a series of gradual shifts—not radical changes—you will be eating better and better (and looking and feeling better, too) over time. We call these shifts the Nine Turning Points, and we're going to show you exactly how to make them a part of your life.

The Nine Turning Points

1

EAT LOTS OF VEGETABLES AND FRUITS.

2

SAY YES TO GOOD FATS.

3

UPGRADE YOUR CARBOHYDRATES.

4

CHOOSE HEALTHY PROTEINS.

5

STAY HYDRATED.

6

DRINK ALCOHOL IN MODERATION (OPTIONAL).

7

TAKE A MULTIVITAMIN EVERY DAY.

8

MOVE MORE.

9

EAT MINDFULLY ALL DAY LONG.

The Body Score Principle

To make it all more manageable, we've devised a helpful tool, the Body Score (see Chapter 10, page 96). It distills the Nine Turning Points into a single, motivating number that you can use to track your progress. The premise is simple: *Raise your score and you'll lower your weight and improve your health.*

As the saying goes, "Give a man a fish, and he'll eat for a day; *teach* him to fish, and he'll eat for a lifetime." This book is designed to do both: In addition to suggestions and prescriptions for what, when, and how to eat, you'll gain solid knowledge and tools that will help you figure out a healthy eating strategy on your own. That means you'll be equipped to achieve and maintain a healthy weight *and* fight chronic illnesses such as cancer, diabetes, and heart disease. Along the way, your appreciation of good food will deepen—and this, in and of itself, will help reduce stress and increase enjoyment. It's a win-win-win fishing lesson!

Most diets will work in the short term, because they cause you to be more conscious about the food choices you make and the limits you set. But most are not designed for the long haul. They tend to be too monotonous, deprivation-driven, or extreme to stick with. And to the degree that many popular diets are all of the above, their effects tend to be easily reversed, leading many dieters into an agonizing loop of gaining, losing, and gaining again—which is as bad for health as it is for morale.

Dr. Willett's Science Bites
Diet and Health—Putting the Pieces Together

TO LOOK AT the impact of multiple facets of diet, at Harvard University we created a dietary score based on a person's intake of whole grains, polyunsaturated fat, folic acid, fish, alcohol in moderation (all good factors), and saturated and trans fat (bad factors). We then calculated that dietary score for each of 84,129 healthy women in the Nurses' Health Study and updated it every four years, when the women filled out a new dietary questionnaire. We found that *women with the highest dietary score had half the risk of developing a heart attack or dying of coronary heart disease during the next fourteen years.* When combined with not smoking, getting regular physical activity, and maintaining a healthy weight, we calculated that a healthy diet could prevent over 80 percent of heart attacks. If this sounds too good to be true, keep in mind that we have known for years that rates of heart disease are more than 80 percent lower among people living in the Mediterranean region, so we are really just advocating what people have experienced with a traditional healthy lifestyle. By comparison, taking a statin pill, the most powerful drug for reducing heart disease, reduces risk of heart attacks by only about 30 percent. (Source: Stampfer, M.J., *New England Journal of Medicine*, 2000)

To make matters worse, many diets can be socially isolating, making the dieter feel like the odd person out a good deal of the time. You need a plan you can live with—and, we hope, live with for a very long time. So we are pleased to present the *Eat, Drink, and Weigh Less* program, designed both to enhance your life and become a central part of it.

What's different about *Eat, Drink, and Weigh Less* is that it's based on the idea of gradual shifts toward positive habits in general, and toward eating lower on the food chain in particular. These shifts are not difficult to achieve because they're not so much about subtracting negatives as they are about adding more of what's good and good for you (notably delightful garden- and orchard-based foods that tend to be lacking in our modern American diets). The more you embrace the *Eat, Drink, and Weigh Less* ideas, the more colorful and delicious your meals will become—and your waistline will trim down in the process. Good habits will gradually nudge out the bad ones, and you will feel and perform better in many ways.

And these shifts are designed with the long term in mind, so this isn't just a temporary plan for when you're feeling bright-eyed, bushy-tailed, and motivated. (We all have days like that . . . but then there's the next day.) These are changes you can incorporate into your life—painlessly and sensibly and at your own pace. What we offer is nothing less than an opportunity for a life-long *positive adjustment to your relationship with food.*

Along with science, there's something equally important going on here: the Pleasure Principle. **Eat, Drink, and Weigh Less is for people who love food.** It doesn't draw a line in the sand with you on one side and good food on the other. The truth is, you can eat beautifully for the rest of your life and be truly satisfied, even as you get healthier and slimmer. Win-win-win! Our guidelines and recipes show you the way to both health and real satisfaction. Instead of starving yourself, you'll eat delicious meals and snacks that will leave you feeling pleasantly full and happy—and sustain your body with the kind of slow-burning fuel it runs on best.

Dr. Willett's Science Bites
How the Popular Diets Weigh In

RESEARCHERS AT TUFTS University recently compared weight loss in overweight or obese men and women assigned at random to the Atkins, Ornish, Weight Watchers, or Zone diets. Over a period of one year, the average weight loss was similar in each group (about five to six pounds), and reductions in blood cholesterol levels were also similar. The percentage of participants who stayed on their assigned diet for the whole year was somewhat lower (about half) for the Atkins and Ornish diets as compared with the other diets. As in most other studies, the amount of weight loss varied greatly within each group; in each group, some participants lost large amounts and some lost none. The large variation in weight loss probably contributes to the enthusiasm we often see about popular diets because we are more likely to hear about the successes than about the failures. This variation also suggests that *one simple plan does not work for*

What Is *Eat, Drink, and Weigh Less* All About?

Eat, Drink, and Weigh Less **is a garden- and orchard-based eating plan centering around vegetables, fruits, whole grains, legumes and nuts, and healthy oils, augmented with a good variety of healthy proteins.**

This is a diet that shows you how to put colorful, fresh produce, whole grains, and other "low on the food chain" items at the center of your plate, regardless of where you get your protein. *Eat, Drink, and Weigh Less* will deliciously deliver you to those five-to-nine vegetable servings a day you've heard so much about. And it's the first major diet that's suitable for vegetarians, meat eaters, and "flexitarians," who look to get their protein from sources other than meat much, but not all, of the time.

Our Promise

Diets are diets. This book is more. Most diets are usually perceived by those who attempt to follow them as something with an "on and off" switch. *Eat, Drink, and Weigh Less* takes you beyond this mentality. Think of this as a manual for lifelong healthy, delicious eating. Whether you follow our detailed weight loss plans or just make our principles a part of your life in a more general way, *Eat, Drink, and Weigh Less* will . . .

- ▶ Guide you through the maze of conflicting information and help you find the positive food choices that work for you.
- ▶ Give you sound, practical advice and inspiration to eat better and get to your own healthy weight.
- ▶ Take into account the real-life demands of your busy world.
- ▶ Fuel your mind and body to improve your concentration, mood, and self-image.
- ▶ Help you fall in love with food again—full-out and without apology—in a fresh, positive way.

Vegetarians *and* Meat-Lovers (and Everyone In Between), Welcome to the Big Tent of Healthy Eating!

Vegetarians with a large or small "v," take heart! If you are someone who prefers to eat little or no meat, you might have felt left out of most diet plans—especially the ones emphasizing increased protein and fewer carbohydrates. These all tend to present a hunk of animal protein as the focal point of most meals, with the green stuff and the high-fiber items relegated to "side" status. *Eat, Drink, and Weigh Less* will help you move vegetables and whole grains to the center of your plate, regardless of whether your idea of a "hit of protein" is savory braised tofu or grilled chicken.

And if you are a confirmed carnivore, but want to green up your diet—gradually and/or greatly—without giving up the foods you love, *Eat, Drink, and Weigh Less* is very much what you have been looking for. We have anticipated your skepticism as follows:

> **Q.** "Mollie Katzen is known as an author of vegetarian cookbooks. But I love meat, chicken, and fish! Will she yell at me and tell me that eating meat is bad, and that I should mend my evil, carnivorous ways? Will I be miserable and deprived on the *Eat, Drink, and Weigh Less* program?"
>
> **A.** No and no! *Eat, Drink, and Weigh Less* will give you a choice of where to get your protein while filling your plate with delicious vegetables and whole-grain dishes. At most, it will trim down the portion size and frequency of meat in your diet, moving it over a tad to make room for more garden varieties. Remember, this is about *shifts,* not radical changes!

(P. S. Mollie herself is a "flexitarian," meaning she eats moderate amounts of healthy protein from animal sources within a broader plan that is low on the food chain. Her recipes celebrate fruits, vegetables, whole grains, nuts, and legumes. And this diet encourages everyone to wholeheartedly embrace these foods while making protein choices from a spectrum of options.)

The bottom line is that protein is important, and so is liking your food. Eating well is about the overall quality and balance of your diet, and the best way to make that kind of balance a reality is to find healthy options that you love. *Eat, Drink, and Weigh Less* is designed to keep you happy, and we recognize that as far as contentment goes, for many people, a little flank steak can go a long way.

SO WHAT WILL YOU GET TO EAT?

IN THE SPIRIT of the Mediterranean region and parts of Asia, you will be very busy chowing down on three good meals and one or two tasty snacks a day. These will include the following.

- Fresh vegetables prepared in a multitude of sensuous ways (more often than not, in a meaningful relationship with extra virgin olive oil)
- Fruit in abundance—fresh and juicy, dried and sweet
- Whole grains in all forms—pilafs, salads, cereals, breads
- Many choices of protein (including meat, fish, eggs, tofu, and dairy)
- Nuts as high-quality snacks and as part of meals
- Beans—in chilis, soups, salads, dips, spreads
- Flavorful seasonings, including roasted garlic, fresh herbs, and fantastic sauces
- Chocolate (yes!) in modest amounts
- A glass of wine (yes!) with dinner (optional, of course)

Our aim is for you to always feel appropriately and happily (but not too) full. Your portions will be measured when you're on the weight loss plan and largely unmeasured thereafter. Once you've reached your desired weight goal, most quantities are determined by, of all things, your appetite. How radical and refreshing is *that* in this age of "cerebral eating"?

How to Get the Most Out of This Book

First, read it cover to cover. Just kidding. We know no one reads diet books like that. But here's a basic road map of where we're headed and how the parts of the *Eat, Drink, and Weigh Less* program work together.

Introduction: The balance of this first section explains how to set your healthy weight goal, and gives you the scientific lowdown on how your body actually gains and loses weight. We'll walk you through the *Eat, Drink, and Weigh Less* Pyramid—our at-a-glance guide to the kind of healthy food choices that form the basis of the diet. And we'll show you how those choices come to life in a quick summary of the Nine Turning Points—the diet's fundamental principles of healthy eating based on gradually moving away from what's less desirable toward what's better for you.

Part One: This is the detailed version of the Nine Turning Points, explaining how and why they work, with lots of tips and ideas for putting them into practice. *We recommend reading this section before you start the diet.* And we want you to know that if you read *only* the Nine Turning Points, use the Body Score Card to calculate (and, over time, raise) your score, and never even look at the diet plans, you'll still have a proven blueprint for weight control and disease prevention that can significantly improve the quality of your life. Put that blueprint into practice any way that works for you, and you can create your own lifelong healthy diet.

We'll also show you how to calculate your Body Score—a tool you can use as a benchmark before you begin the diet, and as a weekly check-in to see how you're doing.

Part Two: Here, we give you a three-stage approach to weight loss and maintenance. Note that you can "mix and match" the following stages, going back and forth from one to the other, depending on your needs and circumstances:

▶ *The Warm-Up Plan.* You can use this as the framework for a long-term, moderate approach to weight control without ever "going on a diet" *per se*. This, combined with the Nine Turning Points and Your Body Score, might be all you'll ever need. The Warm-Up Plan can also be a great set of "training wheels"—a transition program that gets you on the right track in fundamental ways (such as eating more fruits and vegetables and drinking more water) so that when you're ready to start the 21-Day Diet, you'll be primed, and you'll have fewer adjustments to make.

▶ *The 21-Day Diet—A Three-Week Pure Weight Loss Plan.* When you want to "go for it," you'll find the instructions here: detailed daily menus, snack prescriptions, and eating strategies for three full weeks. This is a calorie-managed plan to help you jump-start your weight-reduction adventure while keeping your nutrition and satisfaction levels just where they need to be (and we've counted the calories for you, so you won't have to struggle with calculations). You can "renew" for a second three weeks, and keep going in this very focused way toward your goal (with a few days off in between, if you like) or you can just use this as a springboard and then shift over to *Lifelong Maintenance* whenever you feel ready. In this section, we also present the **Portable Plan**, a simplified option for those of you who lack the time, space, access, or inclination to do anything but run a blender or shove a few store-bought items into a plastic bag.

▶ *Lifelong Maintenance.* This section is for the rest of your life, which can begin right at this very moment, or whenever you choose. We offer simple guidelines for daily meal and snack planning indefinitely once you've achieved your healthy weight goal.

Understanding Healthy Weight

Most of us tend to see dieting as a way to improve our appearance. Going on a diet means eating less to get thin. Thin means wearing flattering clothes and feeling good when you catch a glimpse of your reflection in a store window.

These are great incentives, but it's important to take a step back and look at weight in the bigger picture of wellness. Next to whether or not you smoke, your weight is the most important measure of your future health. It influences your chances of developing a host of serious problems, from coronary disease, stroke, and high blood pressure to diabetes, certain kinds of cancer, arthritis, gallstones, and more.

Eat, Drink, and Weigh Less can help you get to a healthy weight and stay there. Let's start by setting a weight goal that's right for you. One useful way to do this is to look at your body mass index (BMI), a number that takes into account your height and weight to determine whether you're in a healthy weight range compared to a large sample of people. You can calculate it as follows (note that your height is in there twice):

Your weight (pounds) ÷ your height (inches)
÷ your height (inches) × 703 = BMI

Or, just use the chart on page 11. Locate your height and weight, and you'll find your BMI where the columns intersect.

In general terms, a BMI in the 18.5 to 25 range is considered healthy. But take this with a grain of salt. It's clear that if your BMI is above 25, you'd be healthier if you could lower it (unless you are, say, a body builder with huge muscles). But what's less obvious is that even if you're at 23 or 24 you may not be at your healthiest weight. And if you're at a relatively low BMI, for example, 21, you could gain, say, 20 pounds, and still be in the under-25 range, but gaining that much weight would pose clear health risks.

So, think of the BMI as a *range*, not a fixed number like your shoe size. Use it as a guideline to see where you are now, and also to get a sense of what you should weigh to be in the healthy range, if you're not there already. And here's the real bottom line: *If you're within the under-25 range, stay there, and try to keep from gaining weight, even if you have "room to gain" within the range.* (Also, if you have put on more than five to ten pounds since age twenty and are still within the "healthy" range, you would probably be better off if you could shed some of this.) *If you're above that range, a reduction in weight is probably desirable.*

WHAT YOU CAN LEARN BY WATCHING YOUR WAIST

BMI AND WEIGHT-CHANGE during adult life provide two key measures for monitoring your health as you age—measures that have an impressive ability to predict your future well-being, often much more accurately than the high-tech blood-cholesterol measurements that doctors routinely order. Another simple

(continued on next page)

measurement—your waist circumference—is an important indicator of how you store fat, and how that affects your future health. Common sense tells us what science confirms about the negative implications of a large waist size: Someone with a BMI of 25 and a slim waist is likely to have *less fat and more muscle* than someone with the same BMI and a real bulge around the middle. Add to this the fact that abdominal fat has especially bad effects on your carbohydrate and fat metabolism compared to fat stored elsewhere, thus multiplying your risk of diabetes and heart disease. Keeping track of your waist circumference is a simple way to monitor the slow but steady conversion of muscle to fat that tends to accompany middle age unless you consciously build healthy eating and active living into your life. One other factor—osteoporosis that results in height loss—will also lead to an increase in waist circumference, simply because abdominal organs get compressed and need to bulge out somewhere. But if you haven't shrunk significantly in height, an inch or two increase in waist circumference is an early signal that your activity and eating plans need adjustment.

If you are seriously above a BMI of 25, it's not realistic to make getting below that number your immediate goal. You need to lose weight gradually, and ideally with input from a health-care professional, especially if you have diabetes. Aim for a 5 to 10 percent weight loss and give yourself a lot of credit if you achieve that. If, at that point, you are happy with your eating plan and still up for more, aim for another 5 to 10 percent weight loss, and so on.

If you're at the low end of the healthy BMI range and your weight is staying constant, that's great; but if you find you're losing weight without trying to, check with your physician to determine the cause of the weight loss.

How Weight Gain Happens and "Un-happens"

Gaining and losing weight comes down to a simple formula:

Calories in – calories out = weight change

"Calories in" is what you eat. "Calories out" is what you burn. Your body is constantly burning calories—when you're physically active, of course, but also when you're asleep. A 150-pound man, for example, burns a calorie a minute while sleeping. Take in fewer calories than you burn, and you lose weight. Burn what you take in, and your weight stays the same. Take in more than you burn, and you gain weight.

If you eat a balanced diet, based on principles such as those outlined in this book, and exercise about thirty minutes a day, you will probably need no more than around 2,000 calories a day to maintain your weight. Consume 1,500 calories a day at the same or greater level of activity (as you will on the 21-Day Diet), and you will lose weight.

From the point of view of weight loss, *the kind of calories you consume really makes no difference.* That's right. Fat calories, carbohydrate calories, protein calories—they're all calories. Carbohydrates and proteins get turned into glucose, and fat is burned directly. Some of that glucose goes straight into your bloodstream and is used for energy, some is stored as glycogen in your muscles and liver, and what's left gets converted to fat and stored in fat cells to be burned when your body doesn't have enough food or glycogen.

In other words, the balance of eating and physical activity determines weight gain and loss, whether you eat fat, carbohydrates, or protein. And it's the number—not the source—of the calories you consume that determines how much weight you gain or lose.

Now, let's be clear. We're not saying, "Eat whatever you want, because a calorie is a calorie." In fact, we're saying just the opposite: **A calorie is a calorie, so making the healthiest possible choices about where you get your calories is everything. And that's what** *Eat, Drink, and Weigh Less* **is all about.**

BODY MASS INDEX

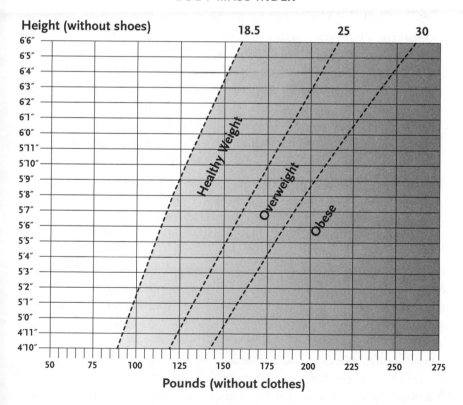

The Myth and Fact of Fat

Contrary to popular mythology, dietary fat (the kind you eat, as opposed to body fat) has never been shown to lead any more to excess weight than carbohydrates or protein. Like any food that contains calories, it can cause you to gain weight if you eat too much of it and don't burn the equivalent caloric amount.

As a nation, we've become obsessed with the idea of "calories from fat." But even a diet that has 35 to 40 percent calories from fat won't cause weight gain if you burn as many calories as you eat. Still, we've been told for years by diets and nutritionists to *cut the fat* from our diets. They're making a mistake, because they don't discriminate between *kinds* of fat. Unsaturated fat is actually good for you (see Chapter 2). Conclusion: If you're trying to lose weight, don't just indiscriminately cut out fat, carbohydrates, *or* protein. Eat the right kinds of each, and burn more calories than you eat. We'll show you how.

Winning the Belly Fat Battle

For most people, belly fat is the target—the body fat they most want to "burn off." But can you actually target specific areas of your body for "spot reduction"? Will countless sit-ups burn away belly fat? And can you lose abdominal fat first, if that's your priority?

You can't really target which fat you want to lose. When you lose weight, you lose it all over. But, that said, it is generally true that more abdominal fat tends to come off first relative to fat in other areas of the body. And it's likely that people who tend to put on fat in the abdomen (especially men) will also tend to lose it there more quickly when they lose weight overall.

So what about all those "ab-building" sit-ups? Sit-ups are a resistance exercise (meaning they involve lifting weight). Like all resistance exercises, they help burn fat overall by increasing your muscle mass. Increased muscle mass means your body burns more calories twenty-four hours a day, even when you're asleep, so it's important to incorporate some resistance exercise, which can include sit-ups, into your regular routine (see page 86).

But as far as abs and fat are concerned, when we talk about abdominal fat or "belly fat," what we're really referring to is intra-abdominal fat—the fat that surrounds the intestines and abdominal organs, *not* the fat that covers your abdominal muscles. To trim your waistline, that intra-abdominal fat is what you need to lose, and it takes a balanced program of diet and exercise to get you there, not just sit-ups.

Now, we're not saying to skip sit-ups and other abdominal exercises. They do, of course, strengthen and tone your abdominal muscles, and the more abdominal fat you lose, the more that muscle-building work will show. Toned abdominals also tend to help pull abdominal fat in—a bit like a girdle—and improve posture, creating the net effect of a trimmer-looking waistline. So the winning strategy in the belly fat battle is: Diet and exercise to lose the fat, plus sit-ups to tone abdominal muscles and enhance the shape of your midsection.

The *Eat, Drink, and Weigh Less* Pyramid—It's the Simple Truth

The USDA created its famed Food Guide Pyramid in 1992 and gave it a complete overhaul in 2005, recasting it as MyPyramid. We offer the *Eat, Drink, and Weigh Less* Pyramid as a more useful, informative, and accurate alternative.

Part of what's wrong with the USDA pyramids is their source: They come from the United States Department of Agriculture, not the National Institutes of Health, the Institutes of Medicine, or the Food and Drug Administration. They're designed, in part, to promote American agriculture, and what's good for agricultural interests isn't necessarily good for your body. Serving those interests while trying to provide impartial nutritional guidance is a tricky task—and the result is a set of all-inclusive, often wishy-washy recommendations that frequently distort the truth.

MyPyramid is riddled with misguided recommendations that ignore evidence about health and diet collected over the last forty years. It's still anti-fat, without sufficiently acknowledging that some fats are good for you. It's not discriminating enough about distinctions between good and bad carbohydrate sources, encouraging you to eat half your grains as refined starch. It lumps together animal- and plant-based protein sources as interchangeable, failing to distinguish between healthy proteins and those that are high in saturated fat. And it recommends more dairy products than you need.

The *Eat, Drink, and Weigh Less* Pyramid is a response, created in the spirit of getting closer to the truth and providing impartial guidelines based solely on scientific evidence. It is a user-friendly tool, designed to give you an instant overview of how the principles outlined in detail in the Nine Turning Points look when put into practice.* In addition to being a weight loss tool, the Pyramid guides you toward foods and habits that have been shown to improve health and reduce the risk of chronic disease.

Just like the old USDA pyramid (and unlike the more confusing MyPyramid) the *Eat, Drink, and Weigh Less* Pyramid directs you to eat more of the foods at the bottom, and less of the ones at the top. We've given very basic guidelines on how often you should eat these foods, but what's important is that you gradually shift toward healthier choices, including getting daily

---

* The *Eat, Drink, and Weigh Less* Pyramid is based in large part on the Healthy Eating Pyramid, developed by Walter Willett, M.D., in *Eat, Drink, and Be Healthy* (Free Press, 2005). See that book for a detailed critique of MyPyramid.

exercise and controlling your weight—factors so important they form the foundation of the pyramid.

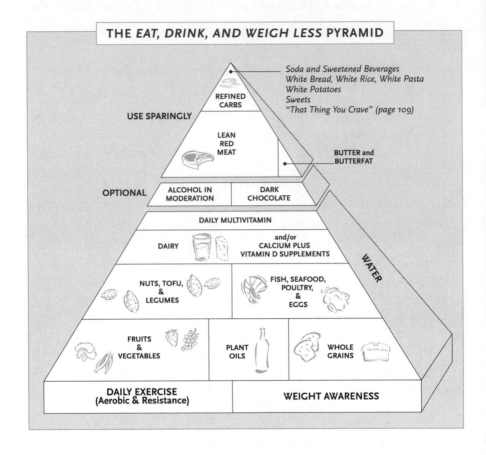

THE *EAT, DRINK, AND WEIGH LESS* PYRAMID

Soda and Sweetened Beverages
White Bread, White Rice, White Pasta
White Potatoes
Sweets
"That Thing You Crave" (page 109)

REFINED CARBS

USE SPARINGLY

LEAN RED MEAT

BUTTER and BUTTERFAT

OPTIONAL | ALCOHOL IN MODERATION | DARK CHOCOLATE

DAILY MULTIVITAMIN

DAIRY | and/or CALCIUM PLUS VITAMIN D SUPPLEMENTS

WATER

NUTS, TOFU, & LEGUMES | FISH, SEAFOOD, POULTRY, & EGGS

FRUITS & VEGETABLES | PLANT OILS | WHOLE GRAINS

DAILY EXERCISE (Aerobic & Resistance) | WEIGHT AWARENESS

The Nine Turning Points

HERE'S A SUMMARY of the principles on which this book and the *Eat, Drink, and Weigh Less* Pyramid are based. They are fundamental shifts you can make in your diet and lifestyle that will help you reach and maintain a healthy weight, and reduce your risk of chronic disease.

1. **Eat lots of vegetables and fruits.** If you don't do so already, try to eat five to nine servings of vegetables and fruits a day. For the most part, they're low-calorie foods that you can enjoy in generous quantities—and they're among the most effective and important foods for health-building and disease-prevention. (See page 19.) Note that, unlike the USDA, we don't count potatoes and French fries in this category.

2. **Say yes to good fats.** Don't indiscriminately cut fat. Eat less saturated fat and avoid trans fat, but *do* eat plenty of unsaturated fats. They can improve

levels of cholesterol and other fat particles in the blood, strengthen the heart against dangerous erratic heartbeats, and fight the gradual clogging of the arteries. And remember, fat isn't any more fattening than other calorie sources. (See page 34.)

3. *Upgrade your carbohydrates.* Instead of simply "cutting carbs," shift from more refined carbohydrates (such as white bread) and quickly digested starches (such as potatoes and white rice) to whole-grain, high-fiber foods (e.g., whole-wheat bread and grains such as brown rice), beans, and other legumes. They'll give you longer-lasting energy and lower your risk of heart disease and diabetes. (See page 48.)

4. *Choose healthy proteins.* Eat more protein from vegetable sources such as beans and nuts—supplemented by fish and fowl—and less red meat and dairy products. You'll consume less saturated fat and cholesterol and more fiber, vitamins, minerals, and healthy unsaturated fats. (See page 58.)

5. *Stay hydrated.* Drink plenty of water, and avoid drinking empty calories, especially from sugared beverages. (See page 66.)

6. *Drink alcohol in moderation (optional).* For most adults (but not everyone), a daily glass of wine—or any alcohol *in moderation*—is actually beneficial to health. (See page 75.)

7. *Take a multivitamin every day.* It can't replace healthy eating, but it's good, cheap "nutrition insurance"—a way to fill nutrient gaps that can show up from time to time, even in a healthy diet. (See page 78.)

8. *Move more.* Getting at least thirty minutes of just about any kind of physical activity a day is an important part of weight control—but it's more than that. Other than not smoking and eating right, it's the best thing you can do to get healthy—or stay healthy—and reduce your risk of chronic disease. (See page 82.)

9. *Eat mindfully all day long.* Eat a nourishing breakfast, lunch, and dinner, and, if necessary, have healthy, modest, nutritionally significant snacks between meals to keep your energy even. Eat slowly, savoring and enjoying your food. You'll feel more satisfied, and you'll probably eat less. (See page 88.)

Welcome to "Food Positivity"

The ideal diet should give you calories that fuel your body in the most efficient, least metabolically stressful way. It would help you reach and maintain your healthiest weight (i.e., a realistic and maintainable weight that is right for *you*). It would give you food that satisfies your appetite both physically and psychologically. It would fit your lifestyle without requiring major shifts in the way you spend your time. And it would naturally—and, for the most part, inexpensively—protect you against chronic illness. Can a diet really do all that? Welcome to *Eat, Drink, and Weigh Less.*

And remember, this book isn't just about dieting—and it's definitely not about starving yourself or making jarring, radical changes in your eating. We're big believers in the psychological and physiological benefits of "food positivity." Every day, we're confronted with so many negative messages about food. This food's toxic. That one makes you fat. It's hard to ignore that scary stuff, and some of it, of course, is true. But all that negativity adds up and, too often, we find ourselves on a battleground. We're on one side, fighting weight gain and unhealthy habits, and on the other side is the enemy: food.

Food is a source of life and joy. And this book is *your* source for countless ways to enjoy the pleasures and benefits of healthy, natural, whole foods. It's also your guide to the science-based knowledge that can steer you to better eating choices. And most deliciously of all, here is your new collection of fresh, flavorful recipes and strategies that will help you feel good, look good, stay well, and love eating all through your life.

The Nine Turning Points

1

Eat Lots of Vegetables
and Fruits

VEGETABLES AND FRUITS:
LOVE THEM—THEY'LL LOVE YOU BACK

No, it's not exactly big news that fruits and vegetables are good for you. You've heard it since before you can remember. But if you can really wrap your mind around this simple idea—and do just a few things to put it into practice—you can make life-transforming differences in your energy level, your appearance, and, best of all, your health.

For starters, many fruits and most vegetables are low-calorie foods that you can enjoy in large quantities. Think of them as a high-volume snack and meal foundation that can fill you up and keep you chewing happily all day long.

But far from being just "diet foods" that can replace something else you might rather be eating, fruits and vegetables are among the most effective and important foods for health-building and disease-prevention. They can reduce the risk of heart attack and stroke, protect against a variety of cancers, lower blood pressure, help prevent diverticulitis, and stave off memory loss, cataracts, and macular degeneration.

Unlike drugs and dietary supplements—to say nothing of items from higher up on the food chain—many fruits and vegetables are, well, dirt cheap and universally available—especially at the peak of their season.

They look great on a plate, not to mention a kitchen counter. And yes, they can be stunningly tasty and satisfying.

If you're somewhat "vegetally challenged," the *Eat, Drink, and Weigh Less* program and its underlying eating strategies will help you get over that, with easy tips and recipes for great-tasting food to eat all day long. If you're someone who's already crazy about vegetables, that's a great start. But many people we know who truly love—and actually *crave*—vegetables and fruits still don't eat enough of them. So, read on, regardless.

The first of our Nine Turning Points is a "more," not a "less." It's an *abundance* recommendation, telling you to *add*, rather than subtract. The message is simple: *Eat lots of vegetables and fruits!* Here's how.

We live in a fruit and vegetable Garden of Eden. Today, in most parts of the United States, even a ho-hum supermarket is likely to stock rainbow chard, edamame (green soy beans), and mangoes. Yet most of us rely on fewer (often, *way* fewer) than a dozen fruits and vegetables week after week—the standard staples we dutifully toss into the grocery cart without much thought as we make our way to the glitzier aisles.

And even after years of "five-a-day" crusading by the National Cancer Institute, the USDA, and others, less than one third of Americans eat five servings of fruits and vegetables a day. The national average hovers around four servings—and guess what? That includes French fries.

So what's going on here? If vegetables and fruits are among nature's most perfect gifts, why do so many of us miss out on their nothing-short-of-miraculous power and appeal? And what can we do about it?

Get Past the Past

For starters, there's the whole "eat your vegetables" stigma to get over—that childhood association with punishment, duty, and deprivation. It haunts us like that plate of overcooked spinach that used to stand between us and dessert. We were told vegetables were good for us. We repeat that wisdom to our children. We even believe it. But too often, too many of us don't really *feel* it.

It's time to step away from the soggy spinach and start a whole new relationship with plant foods. And the first step is opening your mind and simply allowing yourself to consider the possibility that there is more to vegetables and fruits than you realize. Skeptical? Take it on faith for now. We'll show you how and why.

The Labor Issue

Most people, if served beautifully cooked and seasoned vegetables, will enjoy eating them. But getting those vegetables onto the table themselves is another issue. When Mollie teaches cooking classes, her students (all of them food lovers) tend to pose this issue regularly: *Vegetables and fruits are too much work. There's the shopping, the storage challenges, the peeling, the chopping and dicing, the cooking. It takes time, space, skill, and patience.*

Or, barring that, it takes a few good shortcuts. Mollie's students, seemingly to a one, emerge from her classes exuberant about vegetables and fruits. And in her postclass feedback, she never hears another complaint about "too much work." Here are a few ideas that help her students get there.

▶ *Precook.* Do what restaurant cooks do: Partially cook vegetables ahead of time. Set aside a few days a month to shop for, prep, and precook a variety of fresh vegetables. Cook them in boiling water until they're about half done, then rinse them with cold water, let them cool, and store them in the refrigerator in resealable plastic bags. Once precooked, a vegetable's refrigerator shelf life is at least doubled, and it will take up much less space. When it's time to eat, just sauté the vegetable lightly in a little olive oil and garlic, and by the time it's warmed through, it will be fully cooked and flavorful.

▶ *Frozen is fine.* It's okay to use frozen vegetables in many situations (we're especially partial to chopped spinach, edamame, artichoke hearts, and peas)—they can be both convenient and economical. The main compromise here, for some but not all vegetables, is texture, so consider pureeing cooked frozen vegetables into a soup (see pages 168–169). And by the way, the nutritional value of frozen vegetables—particularly those picked and frozen within a matter of hours—can often be better than that of "fresh" vegetables that have been shipped over long distances and stored for who knows how long before they get to your table.

▶ *Overcoming your "knife block."* For many people, what stands between them and better eating is the knife. They simply don't want to deal with cutting the vegetables. Here are some solutions:

  • *Buy a better knife.* Invest in a high-quality, five- to eight-inch chef's knife. The flat-bladed Santoku variety is particularly good for cutting up fruit and vegetables. Keep the blade sharp. You'll be amazed how pleasant prep can be if you have the right tools. Once you're convinced, treat yourself to a good paring knife for smaller jobs, too.

  • *Buy "knifeless" vegetables.* Lots of vegetables don't need cutting. These include prewashed baby spinach, baby carrots, cauliflower (you can break it with your hands), sugar snap or other edible-pod peas, and asparagus.

  • *Buy precut vegetables.* Many supermarkets and produce stores sell prepped vegetables, such as broccoli and cauliflower florets.

They're a bit more expensive, but so is buying a bunch of broccoli and letting it shrivel in the vegetable bin. If paying a little extra to save time and labor means you'll actually cook and eat more vegetables, that's money well spent.

- *In a pinch, raid the salad bar.* If you can't find decent precut vegetables at the grocery store, check out the salad bar. Buy a few cookable items, take them home, and toss them in a hot wok. Expensive, yes, but a great fallback strategy for dinner emergencies.

PHYTONUTRIENTS—HERE'S WHAT YOU GET

A VEGETABLE IS not a vegetable is not a vegetable. How the nutrient content of one tomato, for example, compares to another is a function of how and where it was grown, the season, how ripe it was when it was picked, and how it was stored. But don't worry. There are plenty of common denominators—substances that play critical roles in keeping you healthy, no matter whether you're eating a hothouse tomato or one you just picked in your own garden.

Fiber. Ironically, what you *can't* digest in fruits and vegetables is one of their most beneficial components: fiber. It helps delay the absorption of sugars and fats into the body, reducing spikes in insulin and thus decreasing the risk of heart attack and diabetes. It also relieves constipation and helps prevent the painful inflammation of the colon known as diverticulitis. The fiber found in oats and other grains and seeds traps cholesterol and causes it to be eliminated in stool, thus lowering serum cholesterol and with it the risk of heart disease and circulatory problems.

Vitamins. Science identifies vitamins by studying diseases of deficiency. When a substance is found to prevent these diseases, it is "elevated to vitamin status." Think rickets and vitamin D. More and more research is indicating that cancer, heart disease, stroke, diabetes, osteoporosis, and other chronic illnesses are, in part, diseases of deficiency—and it's possible that the phytochemicals in fruits and vegetables will become tomorrow's vitamins that prevent them. Meanwhile, just think of whole fruits and vegetables as "vitamins" themselves, because their ability to fight these diseases has already been established.

Antioxidants. Deficiencies of a special class of phytochemicals in fruits and vegetables called antioxidants seem to be implicated in the early stages of heart disease, cancer, eye disease, and aging-related declines in memory— and possibly even in aging itself. Antioxidants capture and snuff out highly reactive substances called free radicals, which can cause damage to cells in every organ of the body.

Essential elements. Vegetables and fruits are great sources of elements such as magnesium and potassium that the body needs to accomplish critical tasks, including controlling blood pressure and keeping a steady heart rhythm.

SUPPLEMENTS: WHY THEY'RE NO SUBSTITUTE

WE ALL KNOW that vegetables and fruits are loaded with vitamins, minerals, and fiber. So why not take the easy way out and simply pop a pill that gives us all of that? The answer is both simple and complex. Plants make and store a vast array of compounds that affect our body functions when we eat them. They're called phytochemicals (literally, "chemicals made by plants"). Many of them have yet to be discovered and science is only beginning to pinpoint which phytochemicals—and in which combinations—directly result in the health benefits that we know fruits and vegetables provide. A pill—or even a pharmaceutical "cocktail"—that covered all the bases and contained all the good stuff that plants make would be an enormous discovery. No one can claim to know what it might even contain. Science can't make that pill. But you can. It's a shopping cart filled with fruits and vegetables. By all means, take a multivitamin every day (see Chapter 7). But remember: They're called *supplements* for a reason.

Go from Wimpy to Wow

Who can blame you for not liking overcooked steamed zucchini? It's pretty insipid stuff. But that's not the zucchini's fault. The tastier you make your vegetables, the more you'll eat. And that doesn't have to mean hiding them under a veil of cheese sauce. Turning even the mildest-mannered vegetable into something healthy that you actually want a second helping of is a lot easier than you think.

- ▶ *Try roasting.* Roasting vegetables in a very hot oven concentrates their flavor and brings out their natural sweetness. Throw just about any cut-up vegetable on a foil-lined baking sheet. Drizzle with a little oil and coarse salt. Roast at 425°F, until the vegetables are soft and beginning to brown. For extra credit, drizzle some balsamic vinegar or lemon juice right onto the pan when you take it out of the oven. Serve hot or at room temperature. You'll find yourself reaching for seconds, and probably even thirds. (For detailed instructions, see pages 226–228.)

▶ *The great olive oil two-fer: Flavor and health.* Incredibly good news: Not only are some very good-tasting oils very good for you, but also many nutrients such as beta-carotene (present in many vegetables) are fat-soluble, which means they must piggyback onto fat molecules in order for your body to absorb them. Translation: Drizzle your broccoli with a little olive oil and it will not only taste better, it will be even better for you than if eaten plain.

▶ *Consider the sauce.* Dress your plain, steamed vegetables with an enticing, flavorful, good-for-you sauce. (Yes, they do exist. See pages 191–197.) Or serve one or more of those sauces on the side for dipping.

▶ *Discover nut and seed oils.* Aromatic toasted or roasted walnut oil, pumpkin seed oil, hazelnut oil, almond oil, and so forth are wonderful "finishes" for cooked vegetables. Drizzle on a small amount for a heavenly sensation. Buy small quantities and keep these oils refrigerated, so they'll remain fresh.

Make Salad the Main Event

Poor salad. It's almost universally viewed as an also-ran. "I'll just have the salad," we say with a sigh, as we forgo the temptation of the entrée we really wanted and try to content ourselves with the knowledge that we're doing the right thing. But a great big salad brimming with beautiful stuff and crowned with a modest portion of protein can take you to a whole different place. You'll end up feeling satisfied—full, but not stuffed, light, and energized. The key, of course, is to make that main-course salad really tasty and easy enough that you'll actually make it. Meanwhile, here are a few tips to get you thinking in the right direction.

▶ *Dress smarter.* Ditch low-fat bottled dressings and use one of the six stellar homemade varieties on pages 198–200. This will bring into play flavorful, healthy oils that reduce blood cholesterol and heart disease, and help you absorb the nutrients in your salad. Plus, you'll save money and avoid processed "mystery ingredients."

▶ *Add the right extras.* Small amounts of highly flavored ingredients can go a long way toward making a salad exciting while still keeping it healthful. Try adding a little grated Parmesan or other cheese, or some crumbled feta. Or sprinkle in some lightly toasted nuts. Although these are not usually considered "diet foods," using them as special touches in modest amounts is perfectly fine. They add protein, and something just as important: *pleasure.*

- ▶ *Make "deliberate leftovers" a salad mantra.* Make more vegetables than you need for dinner and drizzle the extras with Mollie's Vinaigrette or Roasted Garlic Vinaigrette (page 198). Store them in a tightly covered container or resealable plastic bag in the refrigerator, where they will marinate beautifully. Then just toss them into your next salad—dressing and all!
- ▶ *Greens—the fresher the better.* The flavor and nutritional value of greens decrease as they're stored. Try to buy salad greens several times a week, so you have a healthy supply on hand at all times. To revive wilted greens, try soaking them in cold water.

Seven Families You Should Know

A single fruit or vegetable may contain hundreds of beneficial compounds, but none contains them all, so it's important to eat a good mix of vegetable varieties every week. Here's a quick reference guide to the most common families of fruits and vegetables. Ideally, you want to include something from each family in your diet every week.

THE FAMILY	WHAT'S IN IT	AND WHAT'S IN IT FOR YOU
Crucifer Family	Broccoli, brussels sprouts, cabbage, cauliflower, collard greens, kale, kohlrabi, mustard greens, radishes, rutabaga, turnips, watercress	Excellent sources of several chemicals that may protect against cancer; folate; calcium; iron; vitamin K.
Umbel Family	Carrots, celery root, parsley, parsnips	Carrots are an excellent source of beta-carotene, which the body uses to make vitamin A. Beta-carotene and related carotenoids may prevent some cancers, heart disease, and Alzheimer's disease.
Melon/Squash Family	Cucumbers, summer squashes (e.g., zucchini and pumpkins), winter squashes (e.g., acorn and butternut), muskmelons (e.g., cantaloupe and honeydew)	Orange members of this class are rich in carotenes, including beta-carotene (see "carrots," above).

(continued on next page)

THE FAMILY	WHAT'S IN IT	AND WHAT'S IN IT FOR YOU
Legume Family	Alfalfa sprouts, beans, peas, soybeans	Excellent sources of fiber, folate, and protease inhibitors (which may protect against heart disease and cancer), protein; B vitamins.
Lily Family	Asparagus, chives, garlic, leeks, onions, shallots	Contain a number of sulfur compounds that may fight cancer.
Citrus Family	Grapefruits, lemons, limes, oranges, tangerines	High in vitamin C as well as limonene and coumarin, which have been shown to have anticancer properties in laboratory animals.
Solanum Family	Eggplant, peppers, potatoes (note that we "disown" potatoes; see "Spare the Spuds," below), tomatoes	Tomatoes contain lycopene, an antioxidant that may play a key role in preventing prostate and other cancers. Also, both tomatoes and peppers contain vitamin C, and red bell peppers are full of beta-carotene.

SPARE THE SPUDS

WE'VE PULLED WHITE potatoes from the vegetable category and moved them to the carbohydrate group because they are mostly starch. Like white rice and white bread, they are easily digested, increasing levels of blood sugar—and, in response, insulin—more quickly and to higher levels than equal amounts of calories from pure table sugar. Studies have shown that potatoes are not linked to the same health benefits as other fruits and vegetables. So we recommend eating them not as a daily vegetable, but only occasionally and in small amounts. But if potatoes are a "don't" (or a "mostly don't"), sweet potatoes (by which we mean both the yellow-fleshed kind and the darker, orange-fleshed variety, which are frequently—though erroneously—called yams) are a "mostly do." In addition to having a higher level of beta-carotene than any other vegetable—even more than carrots—sweet potatoes contain vitamins A, C, and E; folate; iron; copper; and calcium, plus beneficial phytochemicals and a good dose of fiber.

THE VEGETABLE TREASURE CHEST

A-List Vegetables

Go ahead. Eat as much as you want of these—cooked or raw, plain or sensibly sauced, or dipped into something good. When you're hungry, they'll provide plenty of chewing and satisfaction, and adding them will help you raise your Body Score.

Broccoli	Cucumbers
Cabbage	Edible-pod peas
Cauliflower	Salad greens
Asparagus	Bok choy
All dark green leaves (spinach, kale, collards, escarole, chard, mustard, dandelion, etc.)	Brussels sprouts
	Radishes
	Mushrooms
Green beans	Tomatoes
Zucchini, summer squash, and spaghetti squash	Artichokes
	Eggplant
Bell peppers	Jicama
Carrots	Beets
Celery	Winter Squash
Fennel	

B-List Vegetables

These are higher in carbohydrates and calories than the A-list vegetables, so try to limit yourself to one to two servings (½ cup each) per day.

Sweet potatoes	Rutabagas
Pumpkin	Water chestnuts
Jerusalem artichokes	Parsnips
Turnips	

WHAT TO DO ABOUT THE PRICE OF GAS

ADDING A LOT of fiber to your diet all at once can sometimes lead to abdominal cramping and flatulence (or, as we say in medical circles, farting). This happens because fiber is a form of carbohydrate that humans can't digest. It reaches the colon intact, and once it's there, the bacteria that inhabit the colon cause it to ferment. This process generates short-chain fatty acids that are absorbed and used by us as fuel—but it also releases gas that needs to find an escape. Some of the carbohydrates in beans are also resistant to digestion, which accounts for their well-known musical reputation.

(continued on next page)

So what can you do if flatulence becomes a problem when you increase the fiber in your diet? First, try cutting back a bit on fiber until the symptoms resolve, then increase your fiber intake again gradually. Most people can comfortably adjust to a higher fiber intake in a relatively short time. Beano is another handy solution. This over-the-counter preparation contains an enzyme that helps digest carbohydrates before they reach the colon, thus depriving the colonic microbes of a feast of fiber. In formal trials, Beano has been shown to reduce flatulence. It can be helpful as part of a transition to a better diet, but don't become reliant on it or use more than you need, because unnecessarily speeding up the digestion of carbohydrates could partly undo some of the blood-glucose-lowering benefit of these slowly absorbed foods.

Eat in Living Color

When it comes to the nutritional value of vegetables and fruits, nature often makes it easy to spot a winner. There is a correlation between the pigments in fruits and vegetables and the level of healthful compounds they carry. Vegetables with a deeper, darker green pigment, for example, often contain more vitamins than do less vivid ones. Winter squash with a deeper golden hue has more beta-carotene than paler squash. Pink grapefruit brings you more antioxidants than does its white cousin. And there is no contest between romaine lettuce and the iceberg variety. (As Bonnie Liebman of the Center for Science in the Public Interest says: "Eat a whole cup of iceberg and you get ten percent of the U.S. Recommended Daily Allowance for . . . well, nothing.")

When you're shopping for fruits and vegetables, go for variety of color. Get plenty of green, yellow, orange, red, purple, and white. Each of these colors offers unique combinations of phytochemicals, so filling your grocery cart the way a painter loads a palette is an easy way to be sure you're getting a good nutritional mix. Besides, it makes a plate more appealing and eating more fun.

Fresh vs. Frozen and Canned

Because lengthy cooking can damage many important phytochemicals (such as heat-sensitive vitamin C and folic acid), it's important to eat plenty of fresh, raw vegetables and fruits. But you may be surprised to learn that, beyond that, the nutrient content of frozen fruits and vegetables is essentially as good as that of fresh, and sometimes better (see Frozen Is Fine, page 21).

Canning is more likely to reduce nutritional content, as it involves high temperatures, and canned foods are generally loaded with salt, sugar, and other additives you'd be better off without. That said, we wholeheartedly endorse canned tomato products because their cooking process enhances the absorption of lycopene. Ideally, look for the kinds that are packed with less salt. (The brands vary.)

Generally speaking, a canned vegetable is still almost always better than no vegetable at all. After all, until fairly recently, Americans relied on home canning and pickling to preserve their summer harvest, and those practices helped prevent many nutritional deficiencies, such as scurvy.

Conclusion: Keep frozen and canned fruits and vegetables around for those times when you can't get fresh. But for the most part, whole, fresh fruits and vegetables are the tastier and better way to go.

Dr. Willett's Science Bites
Vegetables, Fruits, and Health—the Numbers Tell the Story

PROBABLY THE MOST comprehensive examination of the relationship between fruit and vegetable intake and long-term health was conducted as part of the Harvard Nurses' Health Study and Health Professionals' Follow-up Study. More than 100,000 initially healthy men and women reported their intakes in detailed questionnaires several times over a twelve- to fourteen-year period. During that time, more than 14,000 participants developed cancer, heart attack, or stroke, or died. *Those with a higher intake of fruits and vegetables had a greater probability of remaining healthy. This was mainly due to a lower risk of heart attack and stroke;* participants who ate five or more servings of fruits and vegetables a day had a 25 percent lower risk as compared to those who ate the fewest servings. The greatest benefit appeared to be from eating more green leafy vegetables. Little benefit was seen for reducing overall cancer incidence, although other analyses within these groups have suggested reductions for specific cancers, such as a lower risk of prostate cancer with higher intake of tomato sauce. (Source: Hung, H. C., *Journal of the National Cancer Institute*, 2004)

Don't Forget Cooked Tomatoes

Tomatoes are loaded with lycopene, an antioxidant that has been linked with lower rates of a variety of cancers. Your body has a hard time extracting this substance from raw tomatoes, so cooked tomatoes are a better lycopene source, especially when the tomatoes are cooked with oil, which dissolves the lycopene and helps it enter your bloodstream. The intense heat used in preparing processed tomatoes (such as canned tomatoes, tomato paste, even ketchup) does not appear to diminish their lycopene-related benefits, though much of their vitamin C is lost. Conclusion: Eat fresh tomatoes, processed tomatoes, and tomato products cooked in oil several times a week.

Fruitful Ideas

Fruit tends to fit more easily into people's lives. After all, it's about as simple as buying and eating more of it. Go for the juicy stuff—citrus, apples, melons, berries, peaches, and plums—and, especially if it's organic, eat it with the peel on to get the most fiber. Generally speaking, look for fruit that's heavy for its size and has a smooth, unblemished surface.

> ▶ *Use a knife and a plate.* Sure, grabbing an apple and munching on it is easy and commendable. But if you're not doing that often enough, try a different approach. Use a sharp paring knife to cut the apple in quarters. Cut the seeds out of each quarter, then cut each quarter into two pieces. Put it all on a plate. Now, instead of a big unwieldy piece of fruit, you have a bite-by-bite mini-meal to enjoy, with greater psychological as well as sensual appeal.

A-LIST AND B-LIST FRUITS

The A-List: Best Fruits for Weight Loss

These fruits are low in sugar. Put some or all of them on your shopping list every week, and eat them quite freely—at breakfast, for dessert, and as snacks throughout the day:

Apples	Melons
Berries	Peaches
Kiwi	Plums
Grapefruit	Papaya

The B-List: Fruits to Eat in Moderation

These fruits are higher in sugar or starch and should be eaten in moderate amounts (limit to one serving per day):

Apricots (2 small)	Pineapple (1 cup fresh slices or ½
Bananas (1 small to medium)	cup canned chunks, packed in
Cherries (½ cup)	juice)
Grapes (½ cup)	Pears (1 medium)
Mangoes (½ medium)	

WHOLE FRUIT. No question, it gives you more fiber and bulk, and the process of chewing will make you feel more full more quickly than juice can. Real juice (as opposed to sugary juice drinks) can be an important part of a healthy diet, but remember that it can often pack a major dose of calories. Twelve ounces of orange juice, for example, gives you 168 calories—about twice the calories in an orange—but it's not likely to cause you to eat less of anything else, as a whole orange would. So enjoy juice in moderate amounts (one small glass per day would be a good limit), and try to get most of your daily servings from whole fruit.

Dried Fruit Is Good Food

Fruit doesn't have to be juicy to be nutritious. In fact, dried fruit—such as dried apricots, dried plums (prunes), dried apples, and raisins—can be very good for you. Whether the fruit is dried in the sun or through a hot-air treatment indoors, it retains minerals, antioxidants, and fiber. (It loses only vitamin C and water.) Do remember, though, that a little bit goes a long way, so enjoy dried fruit in small doses.

Five more good things about dried fruit:

- ▶ It's lightweight, so it's a good portable snack.
- ▶ There are many varieties to choose from, so you can keep things interesting.
- ▶ It stores well at any temperature, with little or no spoilage.
- ▶ It's neat—no sticky, juicy mess.
- ▶ It can satisfy cravings for junk sweets and highly processed carbohydrates.

And if you're worried about the intensity of the sugar in dried fruit, here's some good news. Studies have shown that, for many people, blood sugar levels stay low when they snack on dried fruit, partially because the high fiber content slows down the absorption of the sugar into the bloodstream. Look for natural dried fruit that's just fruit, cut and dried, not fruit leather or fruit that is processed with extra sugar. And remember that dried fruit does promote tooth decay, so be sure to clean your teeth and rinse with fresh water after a dried fruit snack.

Getting to Five-to-Nine a Day

Make five servings of fruits and vegetables a day a minimum goal, but aim for nine. It's helpful to keep a food journal until you get the hang of this. A note of encouragement: The greatest benefits of increasing intakes are at the low end. Going from three to five servings a day, for example, has greater benefit than from seven to nine.

▶ *Adding is as important as counting.* Counting servings is a useful way to quantify how many fruits and vegetables you eat. But to help you actually put the five-to-nine-a-day idea into practice, start by adding fruits and vegetables to what you're already eating. Toss some vegetables (this includes minced fresh herbs, such as parsley, chives, or basil) into your scrambled eggs in the morning. Pile sliced vegetables onto your pizza or toast—or into your Very Tall Sandwich (page 155). Munch on fruit and vegetables (raw or roasted) for snacks. Purée vegetables into soups (pages 167–169), add them to broth (pages 171–173), and stir cooked vegetables into cooked pasta.

▶ *Think outside the "square meal."* Most of us were raised to think dinner should include "a vegetable." That was, and still is, a good idea. But here's a gentle reminder. A meal that includes two, three, maybe even four vegetables, is an even better one. Salad can be one of them. So can a handful of cherry tomatoes. If they're prepared in a tasty way, you—and whoever you're feeding—will eat vegetables. So replace that mental "three-compartment" plate with a nice big flat one and crowd it with vegetables. Then have fruit for dessert.

WHAT *IS* A SERVING, ANYWAY?

A "SERVING," in the five-to-nine-a-day sense, is smaller than you might think. It's the amount of fruits or vegetables that would fit in the palm of your hand. For example, it's a medium-size piece of fruit; a cup of salad greens; ½ cup of cooked vegetables, beans, or peas; ¼ cup of dried fruit. It's important to distinguish between a "serving" and a "portion," because a typical portion is often more than one serving. A large salad, for example, can easily count as two or even three vegetable servings.

It All Adds Up to This

Vegetables and fruits come with a natural guarantee. They'll help you reach and maintain a healthy weight goal *and* reduce your risk of disease. A healthy diet is, of course, about avoiding unhealthy foods. But the good news is, it's also largely about *adding* healthy ones. When it comes to fruits and vegetables, that kind of addition can be easy and tasty. In a matter of weeks, you can retrain yourself to see fruits and vegetables in a whole new light—not as "diet items" that replace what you'd rather be eating, but as food you can truly love.

2

Say Yes
to Good Fats

I T'S ONLY NATURAL that most of us see fat as the enemy. It's the evil temptation we feel guilty about eating, the indulgence with which we reward ourselves, even though we know we shouldn't, and the first thing we think of cutting from our diets when we want to lose weight. It's no wonder that, for every food imaginable, someone's come out with a reduced-fat or fat-free version.

Cut the fat, the logic goes, and you cut what's bad. So fat-free cookies and fake-fat potato chips become guilt-free alternatives. As a nation, we're so used to this idea, we spend billions of dollars on these kinds of products every year.

The problem—the wonderful news, really—is that this kind of thinking is wrong. Some fats are bad, of course, but not all of them. Some are not only "not bad," they're actually good for you, and it's important that you *make them a significant part of your everyday diet.*

Take olive oil, for example. You probably know it's a monounsaturated fat and no doubt if asked, you'd agree that it's a healthier alternative to saturated fats, such as butter. You'd be right. But see if the following scenario sounds familiar. You've made some steamed broccoli.

So far, so good. You reach for the butter but think twice and grab the olive oil instead, because that'll be healthier. So far, still so good. But then, you think, "Hmm . . . better no fat at all." You put down the olive oil and squeeze some lemon on the broccoli, maybe a pinch of salt and a little pepper. You sit down and eat your broccoli without much satisfaction, but at least you can feel good that you didn't eat fat.

That's a mistake. Olive oil isn't a "lesser of two evils." It's actively, positively, demonstrably *good for you*. In the context of a balanced diet, you would have been better off drizzling some on your broccoli than going without it. You would have derived health benefits from it, and as a bonus, you probably would have eaten more broccoli—and probably less of something not as good for you—because you would have enjoyed it more.

Which brings us to our second Turning Point. It isn't about the indiscriminate slashing of fat from your diet, but rather about working toward replacing bad fats with good ones. Instead of simply saying no to all fats, you'll learn how, why, and when to *say yes to good fats*.

Fat, Weight, and Health—It's All in the Balance

Since the 1980s, we've been bombarded with messages about eating less fat to reduce the risk of heart disease and cancer. And we've listened. Today, the diet of the average American includes about 34 percent of calories from fats and oils, as compared to 40 percent several decades ago.

But if we've learned to trim the fat from our diets, why, during that same period, has the obesity rate nearly doubled? And why hasn't the war on fat led to a plummeting of heart disease rates in recent years? Part of the reason is that we've cut *all* fats without regard to the *benefits* of unsaturated fats, which can improve levels of cholesterol and other fat particles in the blood, strengthen the heart against dangerous erratic heartbeats, and fight the gradual clogging of the arteries.

But aren't these "good" unsaturated fats still fattening? Not necessarily. It may surprise you to learn that it's not the fat—saturated or unsaturated—in your diet that makes you fat. And, contrary to popular assumptions, you can't control your weight just by limiting "fat calories." The bottom line is, a calorie is a calorie. Eat more calories than you burn—*any* kind of calories, whether they're from fat, carbohydrates, or protein—and you'll gain weight. So, if you keep your total caloric intake and your activity level constant and shift the ratio of the *kinds* of fat you eat to include more unsaturated fats and less saturated ones, you won't gain weight. Add to this a small reduction in carbohydrates, and you'll lose weight.

Another potential problem with simply reducing all fats in your diet is that you're bound to replace them with something else. You do this unconsciously, even when you're trying to lose weight. And for most people that something else is carbohydrates—often simple or highly processed ones, such as sugar, white flour, white rice, and potatoes. Replacing saturated fat with carbohydrates lowers your total cholesterol—though only moderately—but it also lowers HDL (good) cholesterol. Remember, carbohydrates cause weight gain just as effectively as fats if you eat more calories than you burn. And simple, easily absorbed carbohydrates can cause dangerous spikes in blood-sugar and insulin levels that can contribute to diabetes—something that doesn't happen with fat, protein, and slowly absorbed carbohydrates such as those found in whole grains, fruits, and vegetables. So, again, don't think, "Cut the fat." Think, "Add good fat!" And further, think, "Avoid trans fats and shift the fat balance from saturated to unsaturated."

REPLACING SATURATED FAT WITH UNSATURATED FAT: THE HEALTH BENEFITS

SCIENCE HAS PROVEN that eating unsaturated fats instead of saturated fats or carbohydrates will significantly reduce your risk of coronary heart disease and stroke, by . . .

- Lowering levels of LDL (bad) cholesterol without lowering HDL (good) cholesterol.
- Preventing the increase in triglycerides, a form of fat in the bloodstream that has been linked with heart disease, that occurs with high-carbohydrate diets.
- Reducing the development of erratic heartbeats, the main cause of sudden cardiac death.
- Reducing the tendency for arterial blood clots to form.

Unsaturated fats are such an important part of healthy eating that they're included in the foundation of the *Eat, Drink, and Weigh Less* Pyramid (page 14). Make them a substantial chunk of your daily calories and you'll reduce your risk of heart disease. And here's even more good news: Good fats will make your food much more delicious.

Dr. Willett's Science Bites
The Wisdom of the Mediterranean Diet

DR. FRANK SACKS and Kathy McManus, colleagues of Walter's at Harvard, conducted a study among 101 overweight men and women to compare long-term weight loss on a Mediterranean diet including moderate fat content (35 percent of calories from fat) with that on a typical low-fat diet (20 percent of calories from fat). Serving sizes were limited, leading to slow weight loss. After six months, both groups lost similar amounts of weight. But then participants on the low-fat diet began to regain weight and most dropped out of the dietary program. After eighteen months, *the average weight loss on the Mediterranean diet was about 10 pounds (although some participants lost much more), while on the low-fat diet the average weight increased by about 6 pounds. Also, waist circumference decreased by nearly 2 1/2 inches in people on the Mediterranean diet and increased by 1 inch in the low-fat group.* The Mediterranean diet group was followed for an additional year and was able to maintain almost all the weight loss. (Source: McManus, K., *International Journal of Obesity*, 2001)

Dr. Willett's Science Bites
Mediterranean Diet Outshines Low-Fat Diets

TO STUDY THE effect of a Mediterranean diet on risk factors for heart disease and diabetes, a group of Italian investigators randomly assigned 180 men and women to either a low-fat/high-carbohydrate diet typically recommended to prevent heart disease or to a Mediterranean diet that emphasized whole grains, vegetables, fruits, nuts, and olive oil.* After one year, body weight decreased more in the Mediterranean diet group (about 9 pounds) as compared to the low-fat group (about 3 pounds). Levels of inflammatory factors in the blood and insulin resistance, which predict risk of diabetes and heart disease, were substantially improved on the Mediterranean diet as compared to the low-fat diet. This study is consistent with many others documenting that the strategy of *emphasizing healthy fats and healthy carbohydrates improves our metabolic state as compared to an emphasis on overall reduction of fat in the diet.* Better long-term weight control was an added benefit. (Source: Esposito, K., *Journal of the American Medical Association*, 2004)

---

*Please note that this garden- and orchard-based way of eating—and not the unlimited pasta bowl at the Olive Garden or jumbo slabs of pizza—is what we mean by Mediterranean diet.

Good Fat, Bad Fat

Fats come in four varieties, defined by their molecular structure—saturated fat, trans fat, monounsaturated fat, and polyunsaturated fat.

	TYPE	WHERE YOU'LL FIND IT
Eat Less	Saturated fat	Whole-fat dairy products, including whole milk, cream, butter, cheese, full-fat yogurt, and ice cream; red meat; chocolate;* coconuts, coconut milk, and coconut oil.* *Note: The form of saturated fat in chocolate and coconut oil appears not to be a problem when consumed in small amounts (see box, page 40).
Avoid	Trans fat	*Note: Many of the following products are now available as trans-fat–free forms. When in doubt, assume they contain trans fat unless they are labeled as trans-fat–free.* Margarines not labeled as trans-fat–free; vegetable shortening; partially hydrogenated vegetable oil; deep-fried chips or other foods; most fast foods; most commercial baked goods.
Eat More	Monounsaturated fat	Olives and olive oil; canola and peanut oil; cashews, almonds, peanuts, and most other nuts; peanut butter; avocados.
	Polyunsaturated fat	Vegetable oils, including corn, soybean, safflower, and cottonseed; legumes, including soybeans and soy products; fatty fish, such as salmon and tuna. Olive oil, canola oil, nuts, and poultry fat also contain some polyunsaturated fat.

What to Cut

Saturated fat—eat less. Saturated fats are found in red meat, dairy products, and a few vegetable products, such as palm oil. They're solid at room temperature (picture a panful of congealed bacon drippings). Saturated fats increase LDL (bad) cholesterol and contribute to atherosclerosis (artery clogging).

It's virtually impossible—not to mention unnecessary—to eliminate all saturated fat from your diet. First of all, good sources of monounsaturated and polyunsaturated fat also contain small amounts of saturated fat. And studies have shown that eating *some* saturated fat in the right proportion with unsaturated fat is perfectly fine. The point is to move in the direction of less saturated fat and more unsaturated fat.

▶ **Raise your meat consciousness.** If you're a confirmed carnivore, this doesn't require a sudden "cold turkey" conversion. Try to reduce your red meat consumption to a moderate level—say, once or twice a week.

- *If and when you do eat red meat, go for the leanest cut available.* And even then, trim and discard any excess visible fat.
- *Keep red meat servings modest*—the size of a deck of cards or the palm of your hand.
- *Make a moderate amount of red meat the star of a Main-Dish Salad* (page 108).
- *Replace some of the red meat you typically eat with poultry, fish, legumes, soy products, and nuts.*
- *For more information about meat*, see Chapter 4: Choose Healthy Proteins.

▶ **Watch the dairy.** Limit your intake of whole-fat dairy products, including butter, cream, cheese, whole milk, full-fat yogurt, and ice cream. Choose lower-fat versions of these products, but don't be lulled into thinking that "fat free" or "low fat" means "all you can eat."

- *Switch to skim milk or 1 percent.* Of the approximately 8 grams of fat in a cup of whole milk, nearly 5 are saturated fat. The same amount of skim milk has less than one quarter of a gram of fat. If you'd rather avoid dairy altogether, try soy milk. It has more fat than skim milk, but that fat is mostly unsaturated. If you go the soy milk route, check the label—some are loaded with sugar.
- *Use plain, unsweetened yogurt instead of sour cream.* Compare the 48 grams of fat (of which 30 are saturated) and 100 milligrams of cholesterol in a cup of sour cream with what you'll find in the same amount of plain, unsweetened skim-milk yogurt: ½ gram of fat, and only 4 milligrams of cholesterol.

- *Even better: Use nonfat yogurt "cheese."* It's luxurious and easy to make (see page 188), and you can use it as a stand-in for sour cream and cream cheese, or just enjoy it with fresh fruit.
- *Use big-flavored cheeses in small amounts.* Cheeses such as Parmesan, blue, aged cheddar, and feta give you lots of flavor without having to smother your food in saturated fat.

SKIN IS IN

IT'S BECOME COMMON practice among dieters to skip the skin on poultry. But as long as you're eating poultry in moderation, you really don't need to. Cook poultry with the skin on to keep the meat moist. You can remove the skin before serving to reduce the amount of calories you're eating, but from a fat standpoint, it's okay to eat it because it contains mostly unsaturated fat. Fish skin is fine, too.

COCONUT—YES!—IN MODERATION

COCONUT OIL IS unique because it contains shorter forms of saturated fats that strongly increase HDL. We don't really know the effect on heart disease, but when a solid fat is needed, this is a reasonable choice when used in moderation, so don't feel guilty about using it for occasional cooking and for making Thai food.

Dr. Willett's Science Bites
Dark Chocolate Lovers, Take Heart!

DARK CHOCOLATE, UNLIKE white chocolate, contains compounds called flavonoids that may have beneficial effects on the cardiovascular system. To test this directly in humans, a group of Italian researchers fed fifteen volunteers either dark chocolate or white chocolate, about 4 ounces per day, for fifteen days. Then they reversed the type of chocolate that was fed to participants. *While on dark chocolate, participants' blood pressure was significantly reduced as compared to the period when they were eating white chocolate. Also, insulin resistance, an indicator of risk for diabetes, was reduced while consuming dark chocolate but not white chocolate.* Bear in mind, though, that four ounces of chocolate would provide more than 500 calories, so the amount we suggest on a weight control plan would have only modest benefit. Still, knowing that a bit of fine chocolate is nudging you toward better health, rather than in the opposite direction, should be sweet news indeed. (Source: Grassi, D., *American Journal of Clinical Nutrition,* 2005)

THE LABELS OF many fat-free and "lite" dairy products can get pretty heavy, laden with ingredients added to compensate for the richness of fat. Here's a general principle: Be aware of the difference between products that simply have fat removed (such as skim milk) and those that are pumped up with sugar or "mystery ingredients." Food manufacturers want you to believe that you can eat as much of these "guilt-free" products as you want. It's your choice, of course, but consider the possibility that a small amount of the real thing may give you more satisfaction—and maybe even fewer calories—than a larger amount of the synthetic stuff.

Trans fats—avoid them whenever possible. Trans fat is vegetable oil that has been turned into a solid fat (such as shortening or margarine) by heating it with hydrogen—a process called hydrogenation. Used as a substitute for butter or lard in baking and food production, trans fats are a boon to manufacturers and some restaurants, because hydrogenation extends shelf life and flavor stability. That's why these man-made fats are so often found in fast-food French fries and packaged baked goods, such as crackers, breads, cookies, and muffins.

Trans fats (also known as trans fatty acids) are even worse for you than saturated fat. They raise LDL (bad) cholesterol as much as saturated fat, but also substantially lower HDL (good) cholesterol, raise inflammatory factors in the blood, and have been linked with heart disease and the risk of type 2 diabetes. Because of this, the Institute of Medicine, a branch of the National Academy of Sciences, declared there is no safe amount of trans fat in the diet. *Trans fats should be avoided whenever possible.* There is a small amount of a special form of trans fat in dairy and red meat fat, so a little bit of this is unavoidable if you eat these foods. But aim for zero trans fat from partially hydrogenated oils.

▶ *Read the label.* Check the "Nutrition Facts" panel on food packages before buying. Pay particular attention to the labels of margarine or butter replacement spreads, crackers, muffins, cookies, and breads. Look for a trans fat value of 0 grams. Note that some product labels, including those of certain brands of peanut butter, will say "zero grams trans fat," though the ingredients include hydrogenated vegetable oil. This may be because the oil is completely, not partially, hydrogenated, which creates saturated fat rather than trans fat. The increase in saturated fat in peanut butter is small and not of much concern, although natural peanut butter is still a bit better for you. A greater source of confusion is that food labels can say "zero grams trans fat," even if *partially hydrogenated* oils are used, as long as the food contains less than half a gram per serving. While this is better than a larger amount, the best choice would be no trans fat at all (because even amounts of less than half a gram can add up to an undesirable intake). Conclusion: *Avoid anything that says "partially hydrogenated" and look for a "0" in the Trans Fat box.*

▶ *Hold the fries.* Avoid fried foods when you eat at fast-food restaurants. Most fried fast foods—especially French fries and doughnuts—are prepared in partially hydrogenated vegetable fats. A few restaurants, Legal Sea Foods in Boston, for example, are now using trans-free oils for deep-frying, so head for these places when you really crave fried clams. It should come as no surprise that their blind taste tests show that the natural unhydrogenated oils beat trans fats for eating pleasure.

▶ *Don't bake with shortening.* Instead of conventional solid shortening, which contains unhealthful trans fats, use oils rich in unsaturated fat. This may require a little experimentation if you're retooling a favorite recipe. (Note that at least one brand, Spectrum Naturals organic shortening, is trans-fat free. It's sold in most natural grocery stores. More options are emerging, and even Crisco has a trans-free version. But unless you can get these products, your best bet is to use liquid oils whenever possible.)

Dr. Willett's Science Bites
Building a Case Against Trans Fat

FOR SEVERAL DECADES, a small number of people had been concerned that trans fats produced by the partial hydrogenation of liquid vegetable oils could increase risk of heart attack and have other adverse effects. Trans fats were prime suspects because they are artificially altered versions of essential fat molecules that play key roles in metabolism; often a small change in an essential molecule will lead to a new molecule with an opposite biological effect. Although suspicious, the evidence linking trans-fat intake with heart disease was indirect and not convincing. The first detailed metabolic study of trans-fat intake was conducted in the Netherlands by Drs. Mensink and Katan and published in 1990. These scientists randomly assigned fifty-nine men and women to a high or low intake of trans fats for three weeks. On the high-trans diet, LDL (bad) cholesterol rose just as much as on a high–saturated fat diet. However, on the high–trans fat diet, HDL (good) cholesterol fell, which did not happen with saturated fat. *The change in the ratio of LDL to HDL cholesterol, which best predicts risk of heart disease, was about twice as bad on a high–trans fat diet as on a high–saturated fat one.*

Although these changes in cholesterol further raised suspicions about trans fat, they didn't provide a direct link to the risk of heart disease. To study this, starting in 1980, we collected detailed dietary data from nearly 84,000 healthy women in the Nurses' Health Study, and from this information we calculated the intake of trans fat. During eight years of follow-up, 431 women had a heart attack. After adjusting for smoking, physical activity, and other factors that could influence the risk of heart disease, we found that *women with the highest intake of trans fat had a 50 percent greater risk of heart attack* as compared to those with a low intake. As is always important, both this and the study of Mensink and Katan have been reproduced by other scientists. Together, the weight of evidence has led to the clear conclusion that trans fats are guilty of increasing the risk of heart disease, and more recent findings have built a compelling case for their causing type 2 diabetes as well. For this reason, the Food and Drug Administration now requires that trans fats be included on food labels, and *we recommend avoiding them entirely.* (Source: Mensink R. P., *New England Journal of Medicine*, 1990; Willett, W., *Lancet*, 2003)

And Now for the Fun Part: What to Add

Once you've taken a look at the realities of your diet and figured out how to reduce saturated fat and trans fats, the good news is that you get to replace them with tasty unsaturated fats. Monounsaturated fats are found in olive, canola, and peanut oils, as well as in avocados and nuts. Polyunsaturated fats are found in seeds and oils made from corn, soybean, safflower, and cottonseed, as well as in fish, legumes, and poultry. Our bodies can't manufacture these essential fats, so we need to get them from the foods we eat. That's why a healthy diet should include a mix of monounsaturated and polyunsaturated fats.

▶ *Reach for the olive oil.* It's one of the best sources of monounsaturated fats, it's ultra-versatile for cooking, and, best of all, it adds rich flavor and "mouthfeel" to foods. If you're not wild about its taste— or you don't need this particular flavor—look for paler, less flavorful olive oils or use canola or peanut oil.
  - *Swap it for butter.* Get into the habit of replacing butter with olive oil for sautéing, making eggs, and even for drizzling on toast and bread.
  - *Use it in dressings and sauces.* See pages 185–200 for ideas.

- *"Spike" oil with butter.* If you really love the flavor of butter, you can add just a bit to olive oil in the pan when sautéing. You'll taste a distinct butter flavor and, in addition, the olive oil will help protect the butter from burning, so you can cook at higher temperatures than if you were using butter alone.
- *Try this time-honored restaurant trick.* Precook your green vegetables, then reheat them in a tablespoon or two of olive oil with a little minced garlic. Toss in some salt and pepper (page 232).

▶ **Eat your avocados.** But aren't they fattening? Remember: "Fat" isn't "fattening" *per se,* and not all fats are bad fats. Avocados are a great source of beneficial monounsaturated fat, as well as of vitamin E. Add them to salads, a few slices at a time, or mash them merrily into guacamole (page 186). And while you're at it, try these other simple ideas as well:

- *Avocado "butter."* Spread mashed avocado on toast or bread instead of butter. Sprinkle with a little lime juice and kosher salt (see page 187).
- *Add sliced avocado to any sandwich.* Think of it as a natural way to "hold the mayo."
- *Whip it into dressings.* Blend avocado into a creamy salad dressing for use on both fruit and vegetable salads (see page 200).

▶ **Eat nuts. Two billion squirrels can't be wrong.**

- *Try toasting nuts before you eat them.* Toasting invariably enhances the flavor and texture of nuts.
- *Snack smart.* Keep nuts and seeds on hand for snacking between meals. Pistachios in the shell are a great choice because shelling them slows you down and keeps you from overindulging. Yes, nuts are high in calories. The key, when snacking, is to eat modest amounts of nuts *instead of,* not in addition to, less nutritious snacks, such as chips. A small amount will go a long way toward taking the edge off your appetite.
- *Make Super Trail Mix.* Mix nuts and seeds with dried fruit to make a satisfying, appetite-curbing, health-enhancing treat (see pages 175–176).
- *Give nuts a flavorful coating.* Bake them with sweet or savory seasonings (see pages 177–178) to enhance their status as a snack, dessert, or meal component.
- *Toss them on, add them in.* Add nuts to salads for texture, flavor, and substance. Sprinkle them into sautéed vegetables and stir-fries for all the same reasons—especially when you're minimizing meat.
- *Switch to better nut butters.* Instead of typical mainstream peanut butter, switch to natural-style peanut butter and other nut butters made from just nuts. You won't save calories, but regular

peanut butter is generally made with hydrogenated oils that add more saturated fat.

FAKE FAT—NO FREE LUNCH

FAT SUBSTITUTES, SUCH as Olestra and Simplesse, mimic the feel and taste of fat, holding out the promise of weight loss through fat-free eating. But that's a fake promise. First of all, you tend to keep your caloric intake at around the same level unconsciously, whether you're eating fat or not. And in the case of fat-free indulgence foods such as chips, cookies, and ice cream made with fat substitutes, you may even be inclined to eat more, because, "Hey, it's fat-free," so your calorie intake increases. Fake fats feed a fundamentally wrong assumption that all fats are bad. Saturated fats tend to be unhealthy, but unsaturated fats are good for us. What counts is total calories, regardless of food type. *We can easily achieve a healthy diet based on a healthy caloric intake with plenty of delicious unsaturated fat options.* Fake fats are an invention we just don't need.

N-3 Fats: The "Essential" in "Essential Fatty Acids"

You need fat for all kinds of reasons. Fats provide fuel for cells as well as the raw materials for building cell membranes. The body can make most of the fats it needs from any kind of fat in the diet as well as from carbohydrates. But there are a few fats it can't produce. These are the *essential* fats—all of which are polyunsaturated—also known as the n-3 fats or omega-3 fatty acids, and the n-6 or omega-6 fatty acids. Because your body can't make them, they have to come directly from the foods you eat. And you need them. They're beneficial in regulating blood clotting and in preventing heart disease, stroke, and possibly lupus, eczema, rheumatoid arthritis, and a variety of other conditions. They help keep the heart beating at a steady rate, preventing potentially fatal arrhythmias. Because of fairly large increases in vegetable fats in the American diet over the last eighty years, most of us get a pretty good supply of n-6 fatty acids, but many people come up short in n-3 fats.

Try to eat at least one good source of n-3 fatty acids a day. These can include:

Fish (a palm-size serving)—your best bets are firm-fleshed, fatty types of fish, such as tuna, salmon, swordfish, and sardines. But even leaner, white-fleshed fish provides some n-3 fatty acids, so a variety of fish is fine.

Fish oil—for a healthy person, one capsule containing about half a gram of n-3 fatty acids a day should be fine, but someone with heart disease should talk to their health care provider about taking more. Vegetarian sources are also available.

Walnuts (one serving, a small handful)—about 10 percent of the fat in walnuts is an omega-3 fatty acid (this is much higher than in other nuts), which makes them a good source of this essential fat.

Unhydrogenated soybean oil or canola oil (about one tablespoon)

Flax seeds (one tablespoon)—sold in health food stores, these need to be ground and raw for the oil to be absorbed, and they should be kept away from heat, or they will become rancid. So grind them and sprinkle them on cereal and salads; stir them into yogurt or cottage cheese; and add them to smoothies.

Flaxseed oil (one teaspoon)—sold in health food stores. Look for cold-pressed, organic varieties because machine processing can reduce n-3 content significantly. Keep in mind, though, that this concentrated source of n-3 fatty acids is not needed on a regular basis, because dietary sources are widely available and easy to build into the way of eating we describe.

EGGS AND CHOLESTEROL: CRACKING THE MYTH

FEAR OF CHOLESTEROL has sullied the reputation of eggs, shifting the focus away from their positive nutritional value. Yes, eggs are high in cholesterol, with 200 milligrams in each yolk. But they're also very low in saturated fat and packed with valuable nutrients, including protein, polyunsaturated fats, folic acid, and other B vitamins. Studies have shown that adding 200 milligrams of cholesterol a day to the diet increases blood cholesterol only slightly. And people vary widely with regard to how much of their dietary cholesterol actually shows up in their bloodstream. Research has shown that people eating up to an egg a day are no more likely to have more heart attacks or strokes than those who eat less than an egg a week. So keep eggs on hand as a quick, nourishing food to enjoy in moderation—say, about seven a week. (Note that people with diabetes do metabolize cholesterol differently, so for them, limiting intake to two eggs per week makes sense.) And don't forget to use unsaturated fat (or just a token amount of saturated fat) when cooking them.

The Skinny on Fat

Don't just cut fat indiscriminately from your diet, because some fats are good. Replacing the undesirable ones—saturated fat (okay in small amounts, occasionally) and trans fats (all bad news, all the time)—with unsaturated fats is a safe, proven, easy, and, best of all, *satisfying* way to cut your risk of heart disease. But remember that replacing saturated fat with carbohydrates won't do the same thing. Eat one or more good sources of n-3 fatty acids every day. Cut back on saturated fats by limiting the amount of full-fat dairy foods you eat and by eating poultry, fish, nuts, and legumes instead of red meat when possible. And add unsaturated fats by using liquid vegetable oils in cooking and at the table, and by eating nuts and avocados. Finally, don't worry about counting grams of "total fat" or calories from fat. *Just make an effort to consciously shift the balance from undesirable or bad to good.* The *Eat, Drink, and Weigh Less* program and recipes will show you just how to put that into practice and just how tasty the results can be.

Upgrade Your Carbohydrates

CARBOHYDRATES: A WHOLE NEW PERSPECTIVE

Good Carb, Bad Carb

A FRIEND YOU HAVEN'T seen in a while walks up to you at a party. She looks amazing. She must have lost 20 pounds. "How'd you do it?" you ask. "Oh, it was easy," she replies a little too breezily, "I just stopped eating carbs."

Well, first of all, she may think she did, but she didn't. She's undoubtedly been eating all kinds of carbohydrates without knowing it. What she means, most likely, is that she stopped eating bread, pasta, potatoes, rice, grains, and sweets. Why did she lose weight? Practically any diet will help you do that, at least initially, simply because diets make you focus on what you eat instead of just munching away all day without giving it much thought. That means that you're likely to limit your caloric intake, the single most important factor in controlling weight.

And who knows what your svelte friend really did while she was "cutting carbs"? Perhaps she swam for an hour every day, or stopped eating half a pint of Chunky Monkey ice cream every night before bed. The point is, healthful eating and weight management, like life, are never about one thing, whether it's cutting carbs, cutting fat, eating steak wrapped in bacon, or sipping cabbage soup. And some diets tend to want you to think they are. It's easy to set up a villain and then shoot it down.

But remember, in a normal diet, your body converts extra dietary fats, carbohydrates, and protein to fat at the same rate. A calorie is a calorie. And 500 calories of steak, pasta, or ice cream will have the same effect on your weight.

In Chapter 2, we talked about the mistake of cutting fat from your diet without regard to which fats are harmful and which are actually beneficial. The same kind of thinking holds true for carbohydrates. There are better choices and worse ones. And shifting the balance to include more of the right kind— meaning, in addition to fruits and vegetables, grains that are as intact as possible—is one of the most important foundations of healthful eating.

Carbohydrates from grains, fruits, and vegetables should indeed give you part of your daily calories—as much as 30 to 40 percent. But it's important that the carbohydrates from grains come from *whole* grains, which help protect you against a range of chronic diseases. In other words: *Don't just cut carbohydrates.*

The Carbohydrate Roller Coaster: Ride at Your Own Risk

One of the amazing things about how we humans have evolved is that we're able to run on all kinds of different fuels, depending on what's available. Most of what you eat is—or can be—converted to a sugar called glucose. Some of it goes straight into your bloodstream every time you eat and is used immediately by your cells. Some is linked into long chains, called glycogen, and is stored in your muscles and liver. And the rest is converted to fat and kept in reserve in fat storage cells.

Because glucose is the primary fuel for most of the body's tissues, you have sophisticated regulatory systems to make sure your glucose level doesn't fall too low or shoot up too high. As blood sugar rises, your pancreas quickly produces insulin, a hormone that "ushers" glucose into muscles and other cells. This causes blood sugar levels to drop, followed by a decrease in insulin levels. Once blood sugar hits a baseline, your liver releases stored glucose to maintain a constant supply.

Sounds like a pretty well oiled machine, right? Well, it is. But if you abuse any machine, it's bound to break down. The problem is that in a relatively short time, we've changed into eaters of a very different kind than our ancestors were. In particular, modern-day Americans eat more foods loaded with easily digested carbohydrates than ever. On average, we get about half of our calories from refined carbohydrates. And, believe it or not, half of those carbohydrates come from just seven sources: soft drinks; bread; cakes and other sweet baked goods; sugars, syrups, and jams; white potatoes; ready-to-eat cereals; and milk.

These quick-to-digest foods can set off a risky roller-coaster effect. They can cause a sudden rise in blood sugar, triggering a flood of insulin, which, in turn, drives glucose levels too low and thus generates new hunger signals. The sensation of fullness and satiety eludes you, and you reach instinctively for more glucose, even as your liver is releasing it. You're stuck in a loop that makes continuous demands on your pancreas, possibly exhausting its insulin-making cells—which could be the beginning of type 2 (or adult-onset) diabetes. And a diet high in quickly digestible refined carbohydrates can also cause higher levels of blood triglycerides and lower levels of HDL (good) cholesterol, which can lead to cardiovascular diseases.

On the other hand, when you eat more slowly digested carbohydrates, including whole-grain foods, legumes, and vegetables, these dangerous peaks and troughs are smoothed out. Blood sugar and insulin levels rise more slowly and peak at lower levels, and you're less likely to get hungry again as quickly.

FUEL FOR THOUGHT

OUR FRIEND AND colleague, David Ludwig, M.D., of Children's Hospital Boston and Harvard Medical School, likes to describe the body's energy system as a fireplace being set up for a cozy fire. The goal is to get the fire to burn steadily and last a long time. Think of the crumpled newspaper underneath the wood as quick-burning refined carbohydrates and the kindling as whole grains. The logs on top are the proteins, fats, and fiber. If you were to leave off the kindling and the logs and just burn the newspaper, you'd get a lovely initial flare-up, a dramatic flash, and a moment of warmth, followed by—literally—burnout. It's a metaphor worth remembering as you choose carbohydrate sources throughout the day.

Dr. Willett's Science Bites
All Carbs Are Not Created Equal

MANY SENIOR NUTRITIONISTS and dietitians have insisted that all carbohydrates have an equal impact on long-term health. To examine this question, we studied more than 91,000 healthy women in the Nurses' Health Study II* who completed detailed dietary questionnaires in 1991. We used their responses to calculate their intake of dietary fiber and their glycemic index, a measure of rapidly absorbed carbohydrates, mainly from refined starch and potatoes. By 1999, 741 of these women had developed type 2 diabetes. *With increasing intake of fiber from grain products, the risk of diabetes decreased. In contrast, with increasing*

---

*There are two Nurses' Health Studies, and they are both ongoing.

What to Eat, What to Cut Back On

Simple carbohydrates are sugars, such as glucose (sometimes called dextrose), fructose (aka, fruit sugar), and galactose (a part of milk sugar). They give us energy and not much else. *Complex carbohydrates* are long chains of sugars. The main type is starch, a chain of glucose molecules. Our digestive system breaks down starch chains into their component sugars. Another kind of complex carbohydrate, fiber, is indigestible and passes largely unchanged through the digestive system. It's an oversimplification to suppose that all simple carbohydrates are bad and all complex carbohydrates are good. In deciding which carbohydrates to eat, it's more useful to categorize carbohydrates by their effect on blood sugar and by whether they come from refined or whole grains.

There are many factors that determine how quickly a carbohydrate is broken down by your digestive system.

- ▶ *How swollen the starch grains are.* Starch grains swollen with water, such as those in a baked or boiled potato, are more easily digested than the less swollen starch grains in, say, brown rice.
- ▶ *How processed the food is.* Wheat that has been milled into superfine white flour is stripped of its protective coating and broken down into tiny particles, making it easily digested. Quick-cooking oatmeal, which is smashed between rollers, is digested more quickly than "steel cut" oats, which, in turn, take less time for your body to process than the very slowly absorbed whole oat groats from which they are cut.
- ▶ *Fiber content.* The higher a food's fiber content, the more slowly it is digested.
- ▶ *Fat content.* Fat tends to slow down the passage of food from the stomach to the intestine, and thus tends to temper peaks and troughs in blood sugar level.

Understanding Glycemic Index and Glycemic Load

To rate how quickly carbohydrates are digested, scientists have developed a tool called the glycemic index (GI). The index uses white bread or pure glucose (very easily digested carbohydrates) as a standard of comparison, assigning them a GI of 100. For foods with the same amount of carbohydrates, the higher the index, the more quickly and powerfully the food affects blood sugar and insulin levels. An apple has a GI of 55, while mashed white potatoes come in at 102. But here are a few surprises: Cornflakes, sometimes called a complex carbohydrate, have a GI of 114. And ice cream and Snickers bars, which you'd assume to be simple carbohydrates, have GIs lower than that of white bread. The GI, then, helps us see past our preconceptions about carbohydrates and is a more useful distinction than simply "complex" versus "simple."

But the GI doesn't really give you all you need to know to compare foods. Carrots, for example, have a relatively high GI of 131. But to get the 50 grams of carbohydrates used to measure that GI, you'd have to eat about 1½ pounds of carrots! That's where the idea of the glycemic load (GL) comes in. It's a weighting system that multiplies the GI by the amount of carbohydrates in a typical serving. A single carrot, for example, has about 4 grams of carbohydrates, so its GL is 131 percent of 4 (that is, 1.31 x 4), or about 5. A mashed potato, with a GI of 104 and 37 grams of carbohydrate has a GL of 38. A serving of cooked pasta, on the other hand, has a GI of 71 and 40 grams of carbohydrate, so its GL is 28.

But instead of getting bogged down in the numbers, try, in general to cut back on products made from refined grains—white bread, bagels, crackers, and pasta—as well as baked potatoes and white rice. These foods affect blood sugar even more strongly than table sugar. Instead, replace them with beans, vegetables, fruits, whole grains, and whole-grain foods (such as whole-grain bread, crackers, and pasta).

Get to Know—and Love—Whole Grains

Eating whole grains as a side dish is a great way to get past your reliance on white potatoes or white rice to round out your dinner plate. Or try incorporating them in main dishes, tossing them into salads, and using them in place of white rice. Some of them may be more familiar to you than others. Check out the bulk section of a good supermarket, take home a few whole grains, and start experimenting. Making them a regular part of your diet can help you control your weight, fight diabetes and heart disease, improve your digestive health, and keep you off the blood-sugar roller coaster.

Here are the three biggest blocks people have about whole grains:

1. Not knowing where to buy them or how to store them
2. Assuming they are too time-consuming to prepare
3. Assuming they are utterly strange and usually dreary

And here are three easy answers:

1. Buy whole grains in the bulk bins of natural grocery stores, including nationwide chains such as Whole Foods and Wild Oats (these bins are appearing increasingly at more conventional grocery stores as well). Also, many types of whole grains (such as quinoa, brown rice, barley, bulgur, and whole-wheat couscous) are now available in boxes on grocery shelves near the white rice. Or mail-order them via the Internet. Also look for interesting whole-grain hot breakfast cereals (see Shopping Guide, page 264).
2. Whole grains are cooked by simmering them in hot water. They require very little from you beyond your presence and an occasional stir (sometimes). So if you're at home anyway, they will cook themselves on the stove while you are busy puttering with other things.
3. How about interesting, vivid, nutty, chewy, toasty, delicious, and satisfying instead of strange and dreary? They really are!

> ▶ *Precook.* For the same reasons that they're slower to digest, whole grains are generally slower to cook. So prepare them once or twice a week in multimeal batches, and then reheat them when it's time to eat. Once cooked, whole grains will last in the refrigerator for up to five days if stored in a tightly covered container.
> ▶ *Mix and match.* Cook several different kinds of whole grains separately, then combine them. When mixing different grains, aim for a balance of flavor and texture—for example, combining intense, more bitter, chewy types with fluffier, sweeter ones. Experiment! Not only are combinations of cooked grains great as a side dish for dinner, you can add leftover cooked grains to your morning cereal (hot or cold)—or let them *be* your morning cereal (they reheat easily in a microwave). You can also sprinkle leftover cooked grains into green salads.
> ▶ *Accessorize.* Add flavorful ingredients, such as fresh and/or dried fruit, toasted nuts, seeds, milk, olive oil, or other flavorful oils (such as toasted nut oils, which are very aromatic).
> ▶ *Stuff stuff with them.* Use cooked whole grains to stuff poultry and vegetables such as squash or bell peppers.

- *Switch from white rice to brown.* Brown rice and white rice aren't two different grains. The difference is in how they're processed. White rice has had its husk, bran, and germ removed. This makes it less nutritious and more quickly digested. Brown rice has the nutritious, fiber-packed bran coating left on. That's what makes it brown and gives it its nutty flavor.
- *Look for quicker-cooking brown rice.* Quick-cooking (i.e., partially precooked and dried) brown rice products are becoming easier to find in grocery stores. They cook in about the same time as white rice.
- *Discover the "soaking grains," bulgur and whole-wheat couscous.* Bulgur is pre-steamed cracked wheat, and whole-wheat couscous is a tiny whole-grain pasta. Each of these can be prepared by a simple quick soaking in hot water (see pages 238–240)—no cooking involved!
- *Introduce yourself to some new grains.* Wheat berries are whole, unprocessed wheat kernels. When simmered, they have a nice chewy texture. Try them instead of pasta in cold salads. *Kasha* is toasted buckwheat groats (hulled seeds). You can serve it as a pilaf or use it in place of white rice in recipes. *Quinoa* (pronounced "KEEN-wah"), a South American grain, is a nutritional powerhouse and a complete protein.

COOKING WHOLE GRAINS. IT'S REALLY THIS EASY.

Method: Rinse the uncooked grains in a fine-mesh strainer and shake out the water. Place the grains in a saucepan of appropriate size and add the prescribed amount of water and a pinch of salt. Bring to a boil, reduce the heat to the lowest possible simmer, cover tightly, and cook until all the water is absorbed. (It helps to use a heat-absorbing pad under the pot.) Don't peek or stir until the recommended simmering time has passed. If any water remains after cooking, simply drain it off. Or, if the grains seem underdone, add a little more water (up to ¼ cup), cover again, and cook a few minutes longer. For a fluffy result, lightly comb through the cooked grains with a fork to let steam escape. Note: Grains can be cooked ahead of time and stored in a covered container in the refrigerator, then reheated before serving.

Brown Rice (short- or long-grain) *(Slightly sweet and nutty-tasting; perfect as a "bed" for spicy sautéed dishes.)*
1 cup grains to 1½ cups water. Simmer 35 to 45 minutes.
YIELD: 3½ cups

Wild Rice *(Pleasantly bitter and nutty. Combines well with cooked breakfast cereal and with dried fruit and nuts.)*

1 cup grains to 2½ cups water. Simmer 1¼ hours or until tender.
YIELD: 4 cups

Oat Groats *(Sweet, chewy whole grain from which rolled oats are made. A terrific high-fiber breakfast cereal, oat groats are more slowly absorbed than rolled ones.)*

1 cup grains to 2½ cups water. Simmer 40 to 45 minutes.
YIELD: 3 cups

Barley (pearl) *(Very chewy and slightly sweet. Great as a side dish—also good in soup and in Mushroom-Barley Burgers—page 212.)*

1 cup grains to 3 cups water. Simmer 1½ hours or until tender.
YIELD: 4 cups

Quinoa *(A tiny high-protein, high-calcium grain. Mild and distinctive-tasting. Combines well with other grains after cooking. Adds a nice touch to cooked breakfast cereal and is also a good side dish, especially when combined with millet—page 241.)*

1 cup grains to 1½ cups water. Simmer 25 to 30 minutes.
YIELD: 3 cups

Millet *(Slightly bitter, very high in protein. Good for breakfast with milk and honey. Also combines well with quinoa as a side dish—page 241.)*

1 cup grains to 1½ cups water. Simmer 25 to 30 minutes.
YIELD: 3 cups

Buckwheat Groats *(Pungent and nutty. Also known as kasha and best known as the star of the East European–style classic, Kasha Varnishkes—page 242.)*

1 cup grains to 1½ cups water. Simmer 10 minutes.
YIELD:: 3½ cups

Cracked Wheat *(Sweet and earthy. Not really a whole grain, as it is, literally, cracked. Included here because it makes a great breakfast cereal. Note: This is similar to bulgur, except it is not pre-steamed.)*

1 cup grains to 2 cups water. Simmer 10 minutes.
YIELD: 3 cups

Amaranath *(Glutinous and sweet, it becomes the consistency of porridge when cooked. So consider serving amaranath for breakfast either with, or as, your cooked cereal.)*

1 cup grains to 1¾ cups water. Simmer 25 minutes.
YIELD: 2 cups

(continued on next page)

Wheat Berries *(Very chewy. Slightly sweet and earthy. A wonderful highly textured addition to soups, salads, and side dishes.)*

1 cup grains to 2 cups water. Simmer 2 to 2½ hours—longer for red (hard) wheat and shorter for white (soft) wheat.

YIELD: 3 cups

Spelt *(Very chewy. Slightly sweet and earthy. An ancient form of wheat. Similar uses to wheat berries.)*

1 cup grains to 1½ cups water. Simmer 50 to 60 minutes.

YIELD: 2 cups

Kamut *(Similar to spelt. Another ancient form of wheat. Similar uses to wheat berries.)*

1 cup grains to 2½ cups water. Simmer 1¼ hours.

YIELD: 2½ cups

Rye Berries *(Seriously chewy and pleasantly bitter. Combines well with sweeter grains, cooked separately. Very savory as a side dish.)*

1 cup grains to 2½ cups water. Simmer 1½ hours.

YIELD: 2½ cups

So What Is a Whole-Grain Food?

Whole-grain foods are made with significant amounts of whole grains or whole-grain flours. But food packaging and marketing gimmicks tend to make identifying true whole-grain foods in the grocery store harder than it should be. Many products that look like whole-grain foods aren't. Check food labels before you buy. "Wheat flour" is not an indication that a product is made with whole grains, since even the most refined white flour can still be called wheat flour. A lovely slice of brown bread might be a whole-wheat impostor, deriving its earthy hue from molasses (or something worse) rather than from whole grains. And, generally speaking, if a product made with whole-grain flour is a better choice than one made with refined white flour, one made with intact or coarsely milled kernels is even better, because it will be more slowly digested.

Look for the word "whole" in the ingredient statement (as in "whole wheat," "whole oats," "whole rye," etc.), and make sure that the whole grain appears relatively high—if not first—on the ingredient list. Products that boast "made with whole grains" on their packages may turn out to be *mostly* made with *refined grains*. Checking the relative position of the whole grains on the ingredient statement is the best way to determine if a product is a good whole-grain source. (See the Shopping Guide beginning on page 264.)

Eat More Whole-Grain Foods—Here's How

Whether you buy whole grains, whole-grain flours, or products made with either, here are some easy ways to put them on your table and welcome them into your life.

- ▶ *Wake up to whole grains.* Have a bowl of whole-grain cereal—such as steel-cut oats —for breakfast. (See Shopping Guide, page 266.) Or switch to a cold cereal that lists whole wheat, oats, or other grains first on the ingredient statement (or, as a second-best option, quick-cooking or instant oatmeal, which your body breaks down more quickly).
- ▶ *When you break bread, make it whole-grain.* Look for breads whose first ingredient includes the word "whole." (See Shopping Guide, pages 264–265.) More and more whole-grain bread options—from pitas to tortillas—are now available.
- ▶ *Consider whole-wheat pasta.* As the benefits of whole grains become more talked about, whole-wheat pasta is showing up in more supermarkets. The Italian import, De Cecco, is particularly good, and the Barilla brand has now added a whole-grain line. In general, whole-wheat pasta is a bit heavier and chewier (and more filling), so try it with heartier sauces, with which its earthy flavor will be more at home.
- ▶ *Use whole-grain flours for baking.* Experiment with substituting up to half the refined white flour you use in baking with whole-wheat or other whole-grain flours (available in natural foods groceries). The result may be a bit denser, but you'll also get the benefit of a nuttier, more complex flavor.

More of What's Good

Are you starting to notice a pattern? The *Eat, Drink, and Weigh Less* program is about shifting your priorities and paradigms. It's about adding more of what's good for you. More vegetables and fruits. More unsaturated fats instead of saturated. And more whole-grain foods, beans, and legumes instead of refined carbohydrates. Again, think directionally, not numerically. And instead of just cutting carbs, make conscious choices that tip the balance toward health. Take a look at Parts Three and Four to see how that translates into day-to-day eating. Then call your svelte friend who got that way on a "low-carb" diet, and tell her you're just sitting down to a nice plate of scrumptious whole-wheat pasta with fresh tomato-basil sauce.

4

Choose
Healthy Proteins

PROTEINS: GO FROM HUNTER TO GATHERER

Meat, yes! Meat, no! Soy, yes! Soy, no! Every day, it seems, there's a new diet and a new diatribe to reckon with. Well, by now we hope it comes as no surprise that we want you to cut through all the conflicting information and simply make sensible choices and consume moderately.

Just as we did with vegetables, fruits, fat, and carbohydrates, when it comes to protein, we advocate a shift *toward* new foods, as opposed to prohibitions that take food *away*. If you think about protein, you probably think first about meat and dairy. The *Eat, Drink, and Weigh Less* program is neither vegetarian nor vegan (although vegetarians and vegans can find plenty to eat here). It is what some people call "flexitarian," that is, largely plant-based, with moderate amounts of protein from animal sources, if desired. Here's our basic philosophy: *Eat more protein from vegetable sources such as beans and nuts—supplemented by fish and fowl—and less red meat and dairy products.* In other words, shift from "hunter" proteins to "gatherer" ones.

The biggest question this raises for people is, "Will the *Eat, Drink, and Weigh Less* program give me enough protein?" The short answer is, "Absolutely."

Just how much protein *is* enough? You need to take in about 8 grams of protein daily for every 20 pounds of your body weight. That works out to about 50 grams of protein a day for an average woman and 65 grams for an average man. Because protein is abundant in so many of the foods that we normally eat, you can hit that goal pretty easily. A cup of low-fat yogurt has 11.9 grams of protein. A 6-ounce serving of roast chicken has 42.5 grams. Together, that comes to around 55 grams. A vegan-vegetarian version of this, over the course of a day, might be 8 ounces of nigari tofu (40 grams of protein), a cup of wild rice (7 grams), and a cup of cooked chickpeas (12 grams).

Check out the chart on the following pages, and you'll see just how much protein is found in a typical serving of the most common sources. You'll also see that the ones that offer you the most protein per ounce are animal sources. But it doesn't follow that they should necessarily be your default proteins. *Eat, Drink, and Weigh Less* doesn't forbid them, it simply suggests that you eat them in moderate amounts and get most of your protein from "gatherer" sources. What matters is less the source of the protein (animal or vegetable), and more the total *protein package* that a food offers. Red meat is a great source of protein. Unfortunately, it's also a great source of saturated fat and cholesterol. The same is true for whole milk or dairy products made from whole milk.

So, if you love red meat, choose the leanest cuts you can find, and don't go for huge amounts. About two servings of red meat a week, each about the size of the palm of your hand (or roughly 4 ounces each, if you prefer to think of it that way), in the context of a balanced diet and exercise, is generally just fine. Chicken, turkey, and fish are better options, and you can have slightly larger portions than of beef. Beans, nuts, grains, and other vegetable sources are excellent, because they're low in saturated fat and high in fiber. We don't usually think of grains as being protein sources because the amount per serving is modest, but they can contribute importantly to overall intake when they are consumed at most meals.

WHAT PROTEIN IS, AND WHAT IT DOES

PROTEINS ARE LONG chains made from twenty or so building blocks called amino acids. Your body makes proteins constantly, and because you don't store amino acids, as you do fats, you need a near-daily supply of protein. Your hair, skin, and muscles, the hemoglobin in your blood, and the many enzymes that keep you alive—all of these are mostly protein. In fact, protein is the basic structural unit of our bodies. Proteins regulate fluid balance and are major components of many hormones, and of antibodies that fight infection. They transport nutrients in the bloodstream and are essential to the bone structure and to the health, maintenance, and repair of muscle tissue.

RANKING COMMON DIETARY PROTEIN SOURCES

FOOD	SERVING SIZE	PROTEIN (GRAMS)	APPROX. % DAILY VALUE*	CALORIES
Lean hamburger (10% fat)	4 oz.	32.4	65	301
Vegetarian burger patty	3 oz.	10	21	70–90
Tempeh, cooked	4 oz.	21	42	223
Seitan	3 oz.	30	62	140
Roast chicken	6 oz.	42.5	85	284
Fish	6 oz.	41.2	82	190
Tuna, light, water packed, drained	6 oz.	44	86	198
Beefsteak, broiled	4 oz.	32	63	364
Cottage cheese, 1% butterfat	1 cup	28	56	163
Low-fat yogurt	8 oz.	11.9	24	144
Tofu, firm	6 oz.	20	42	240
Tofu, silken, firm (Mori-Nu)	4 oz.	7	14	62
Edamame	½ cup	11	22	126
Lentils, cooked	½ cup	9	18	115
Skim milk	1 cup	8.4	17	86
Whole milk	1 cup	8	16	150
Split peas, cooked	½ cup	8.1	16	115
Kidney beans, cooked	½ cup	7.6	15	112
Peanuts, dry roasted	1 oz. (¼ cup)	7.5	15	165
Cheddar cheese	1 oz. or 1-inch cube	7.1	14	114
Macaroni, cooked	1 cup	6.8	13	197
Soy milk	1 cup	6.7	13	81
Egg	1 large	6.3	12+	78

FOOD	SERVING SIZE	PROTEIN (GRAMS)	APPROX. % DAILY VALUE*	CALORIES
Almonds, dry roasted	1 oz. (¼ cup)	6	12	172
Whole-wheat bread	2 oz. (2 slices)	6	12	138
White bread	2 oz. (2 slices)	4	10	160
Rice, white, short grain, cooked	1 cup	4.4	9	242
Rice, white, med. grain, cooked	1 cup	4.4	9	242
Rice, white, long grain, cooked	1 cup	4.2	8	205
Rice, brown, med. grain, cooked	1 cup	4.5	9	218
Rice, brown, long grain, cooked	1 cup	5	10	216
Barley, pearl, cooked	1 cup	3.5	7	193
Quinoa, cooked	½ cup	6	12	128
Walnuts	1 oz. (¼ cup)	4.3	8	185
Broccoli, cooked	5-inch piece	4.2	8	39
Baked potato	2 x 5 inches	3	6	145
Corn, cooked	1 ear	2.6	5	83

*Based on Daily Value ("DV") for protein of 50 grams in a 2,000-calorie diet.

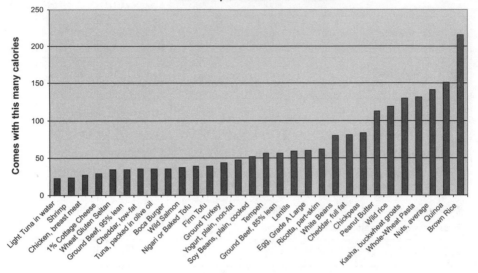

Calories per 5 Grams of Protein

Comes with this many calories (y-axis, 0 to 250)

5 grams of protein in these foods (x-axis):
Light Tuna in water, Shrimp, Chicken, breast meat, 1% Cottage Cheese, Wheat Gluten Seitan, Ground Beef, 95% lean, Cheddar, low-fat, Tuna, packed in olive oil, Boca Burger, Wild Salmon, Nigari or Baked Tofu, Firm Tofu, Ground Turkey, Yogurt, plain, non-fat, Soy Beans, plain, cooked, Tempeh, Ground Beef, 85% lean, Lentils, Egg, Grade A Large, Ricotta, part-skim, White Beans, Cheddar, full fat, Chickpeas, Peanut Butter, Wild rice, Kasha, buckwheat groats, Whole-Wheat Pasta, Nuts, average, Quinoa, Brown Rice

---

AN IDEA YOU CAN HOLD IN THE PALM OF YOUR HAND

AN EASY WAY to measure a serving of protein is to imagine fitting it in the palm of your hand. The bigger you are, of course, the bigger your palm is, which means you get a slightly bigger serving size.

Nutrition Starts with "N-U-T"

Not only are nuts not junk food, they're a great source of protein and further nutritional goodness. An ounce of almonds, walnuts, peanuts, or pistachios gives you about 8 grams of protein, the same as a glass of milk. Nuts do contain large amounts of fat, but it's mostly unsaturated fat, which reduces LDL (bad) cholesterol and keeps HDL (good) cholesterol high.

Several studies have shown that eating nuts (and seeds, which contain similar good protein and healthy fat) on most days of the week can greatly reduce the risk of heart attack and heart disease. Just remember to eat them as a *replacement* for junk food or less healthy snacks, *not in addition to* these foods.

▶ *Turn them into dips or sauces.* The toasty richness of nuts and seeds can greatly enhance vegetable snacks. Try dipping raw vegetables into any kind of nut butter. Also, spoon Tahini Sauce (page 191) over cooked vegetables or grains.

- ▶ *Add them to salads.* Toasted nuts give the gift of crunch, interest, and extra nutritional value to salads.
- ▶ *Try a new nut butter.* Various nut- and seed-based butters are becoming more widely available. If you're not partial to peanut butter, try something new. At a good health-oriented grocery store, you can find everything from almond and cashew to hazelnut and macadamia butters.

Dr. Willett's Science Bites

Peanut Butter—Spreading the Good News

WHEN WE THINK of protein, red meat, eggs, and chicken often come to mind. But peanuts and peanut butter can also be a good source of protein, and, when spread on whole-grain bread, can be a quick, economical, and tasty lunch (add a bit of low-sugar jam if you're looking for variety). We examined the relation between consumption of peanuts and peanut butter and risk of type 2 diabetes among more than 83,000 women over a period of sixteen years in the Nurses' Health Study. During this time, 3,206 participants developed diabetes. *Women who consumed peanut butter five or more times per week had a 21 percent lower risk of developing diabetes* as compared to those who almost never ate peanut butter; consumption of whole nuts was also associated with lower risk. In contrast, we have consistently seen *increased risks of diabetes with higher consumption of bologna, hot dogs, and other processed meats.* Thus, replacing these meats with a peanut butter sandwich provides a double win for health. And while the question of calories in nuts is often raised, in this study and most others, *people who consume nuts regularly tend to weigh a bit less, not more,* than those who do not, probably because nuts dampen hunger for many hours. (Source: Jiang, R., *Journal of the American Medical Association,* 2003)

Getting Complete Proteins

Some dietary proteins are complete—they contain all the amino acids needed for your body to make new protein. Others are incomplete, meaning that they lack one or more essential amino acids, which your body can't produce. Meat, poultry, fish, eggs, and dairy tend to be good sources of complete proteins, while vegetable protein is often incomplete. So, the more you shift away from animal sources and toward plant ones, the more important it is to choose combinations of foods that complement one another (such as rice and beans, peanut butter and whole-grain bread, tofu and brown rice)—and to eat a good mix of beans, nuts, grains, and vegetables to ensure that no essential components of protein are missing.

A Note to Vegetarians and Vegans

The lower you go on the food chain—as you move from "hunter" to "gatherer"—the more you need to think about whether you're getting enough protein. If you are a lacto-ovo vegetarian, and you consume modest amounts of cottage cheese, low-fat milk, and eggs on a regular basis, and also include in your daily diet healthy portions of soy products (such as tofu and tempeh), beans, whole grains, and regular, smaller servings of nuts, you should have no problem getting enough protein.

And if you are a vegan, here's what a day's worth of protein looks like (based on about 55 grams of protein per day):

TWO SAMPLE DAILY
PROTEIN PLANS FOR VEGANS

Plan One

    3 oz. cooked seitan (see page 210)—very high "gatherer protein" marks!

    6 ounces baked—or nigari—tofu (see pages 204–205)

    1 cup cooked quinoa (see page 55)

    ¼ cup almonds

Plan Two

    6 ounces cooked tempeh (see page 209)

    2 tablespoons peanut butter

    1 cup cooked kasha (buckwheat groats) (see page 55)

    1 cup cooked beans

Enjoy the above along with five to nine servings of fruits and vegetables each day. Vegans should also note that they need to supplement their diets with nutrients that are part of the typical animal protein package, especially vitamin B_{12}, which can be obtained through a standard multivitamin.

Soy: Good, but Not a Silver Bullet

Protein from soy foods, such as tofu and soy milk, is a very good alternative to animal protein, but that doesn't mean you should consume it in huge quantities. Research has shown that soy foods can lower cholesterol, but you would need to eat very large amounts to see that benefit. Soy foods also contain powerful biological agents called phytoestrogens. Because some studies have suggested that high intakes may increase risks of breast cancer (but other studies suggest reduced risk), we recommend soy foods in moderation.

Three to four servings of soy-based products a week is a good target—and that can be higher (up to one serving a day) for vegans and vegetarians. If your family is from East Asia and your traditional diet includes several modest servings of soy a day, there is no need to change this pattern.

Protein in Practice

Most of us get enough protein. Although vegans need to be sure they get enough and have a variety of sources, other people, unless they're on a very extreme diet, don't need to be concerned about counting protein grams. For most people, the question to keep in mind is not *how much* but *from what source*.

So, here's our protein point of view: *Keep it varied, and aim for at least 50 percent plant-based.* Happy gathering!

5

Stay Hydrated

THE ANSWER IS CLEAR AS WATER

WE HUMANS LOOK pretty solid. But more than half of our body weight is actually liquid—a briny fluid, much like the seawater that first nourished all primordial life. That fluid keeps us in good working order, cushioning and hydrating our cells, tissues, and organs, transporting nutrients, and eliminating waste from the body. So it's really only half true that you are what you eat: You're also *what you drink*.

Fluid In, Fluid Out

In order to maintain a constant temperature and to dispose of waste, your body loses about half a gallon of liquid every day through sweat, exhaled air, and urine. On a hot day, you lose even more. Exercise vigorously, and you sweat off up to an additional quart of liquid an hour. And it all needs to be replaced.

When your body fluids are depleted, you become dehydrated. Extreme dehydration is not a concern if your diet is reasonably balanced, your activity level is not excessive, and you're not stranded in a desert. But minor dehydration is sneakier, because it's not always easy to spot. It can make you feel grumpy and tired and make it hard to concentrate. And if it becomes chronic, it can cause constipation and may even lead to kidney stones and bladder cancer.

Minor dehydration can be avoided easily by drinking enough fluids throughout the day. But if you tend to drink liquids only when you're thirsty, you may not be drinking enough of them. Thirst does help you gauge your level of hydration, but it's not quite as reliable a guide as you might assume. By the time you actually feel thirsty, your fluid level can often already be too low, and as you age, your sense of thirst tends to become an even less dependable indicator of dehydration.

It's also important to recognize that thirst and hunger are both physiologically and psychologically driven. When you feel hungry between meals, what you may be experiencing is dehydration. In other words, when you think you're hungry what you may be—even though you don't realize it—is thirsty. But you reach for food without much thought and wind up overeating. Much of what the *Eat, Drink, and Weigh Less* program is about is being conscious of how you respond to cues of hunger and thirst throughout the day. The next time you feel a little hungry, try reaching for a glass of water. You may be surprised that the refreshment it brings you turns off that hunger switch until your next meal.

In general, your best bet is to just stay hydrated, regardless of how thirsty or hungry you feel, instead of waiting for cues from your body. How hydrated? Well, you need about a milliliter of fluid for every calorie you burn. That works out to about 64 ounces (8 cups) of liquid a day for a 2,000-calorie-a-day diet. Some of that liquid can come from food and the rest can come from pretty much any beverage at all. Drink a glass of something liquid between meals and a glass with each meal, and, if you follow the basic guidelines of the *Eat, Drink, and Weigh Less* program, you'll have no problem staying hydrated.

But, that said, just as with fats, carbohydrates, and proteins, with liquids some choices are smarter than others. The good news is that the beverage at the top of the smart list is ubiquitous, inexpensive, thirst-quenching, and easy to love. You guessed it: water.

When it comes to hydration, water has 100 percent of what you need, with no calories or additives. And at less than a penny a glass (or, if you buy it bottled, still often less than you'd pay for lemonade or soda), it's a bargain that's hard to beat—especially when you compare it to the alternatives.

A Look at Liquid Options

Remember our bottom-line truth: A calorie is a calorie. Drink water and you hydrate without adding calories. Drink regular soda or juice and you're increasing your caloric intake. But, if you're like most people, chances are you see "liquid calories" as somehow different from "food calories," if you make note of them at all—and that's a big if. So you may not be compensating for the calories you drink by eating less. Let's look at a few of the most common beverage options in this light.

Sodas. Just how popular is pop? Sodas make up a staggering 25 percent of the liquids Americans drink. If you asked people how many teaspoons of sugar they wanted in their tea and they said, "Oh . . . seven, maybe eight," you'd assume they were either crazy or six years old. But that's how much sugar you'll find in a typical 12-ounce can of soda. And who drinks just 12 ounces anymore, when that's a "small" at most fast-food places?

The problem, of course, is that sodas deliver pure calories with no nutritional value. A soda a day may not sound like much, but if you didn't eat less to compensate for its 150 calories, you could gain 15 pounds in a year!

And even if you *do* eat less or exercise more to make room for that daily soda, there's the sugar issue. Taking in a megadose of rapidly digestible simple sugars in the relatively short time it takes to guzzle a soda triggers rapid, intense spikes in blood sugar and insulin, which, over time, may lead to diabetes and may also reduce blood levels of HDL (good) cholesterol and raise blood levels of triglycerides, increasing the risk of heart disease.

So, what about calorie-free sodas? They're a better choice than the sugared kind, but still an expensive way to get water. The sugar substitutes they use (such as saccharin, aspartame, and sucralose) probably don't present much of a health hazard, but the jury is still out about their effect on children who may consume large amounts of them over a lifetime. Diet sodas are artificially sweetened water. You're better off drinking the natural version—flavored, if you like, with a twist of lemon or maybe a splash of juice, or brewed as an herbal iced tea.

▶ *So long, soda.* If you're a habitual soda drinker—at the level of one can a day or more—try this one-month experiment: Buy a case or two of single-serve bottles of sparkling water. Use them to replace the sodas in your home and office fridges. Choose waters flavored with citrus, if you like, as long as they don't contain sugar. Reach for a sparkling water when the craving for soda hits. Opening the cap and holding a cool beverage in your hand will help, in a modest way, to satisfy your beverage urge. After a month, you're likely to experience fewer soda cravings, and, if nothing else, to be much more conscious of them. If you can replace your soda habit with a water habit, you'll stay hydrated and take in fewer empty calories every day.

Sodas and Sugared Drinks—"Waisted" Calories

IN THE UNITED STATES, a large percentage of carbohydrates are consumed in the form of sodas and fruit drinks or fruit punch, which are all mainly sugar solutions. Sugar in fluid form seems to be all too easy to consume and the calories barely register in our control system that helps us unconsciously regulate appetite. Because the effect of these beverages on body weight has been a matter of dispute, we examined this issue in the Nurses' Health Study II. *Women who increased their intake of soda or fruit punch over a four-year period gained weight, and those who reduced their intake lost weight.* Also, during eight years of follow-up, *women who consumed one soda or glass of fruit punch per day had a nearly two-fold higher risk of type 2 diabetes* as compared to those who rarely consumed these beverages. This double whammy is reason enough to make consumption of sugared beverages, at most, an infrequent indulgence. (Source: Shulze, M., *Journal of the American Medical Association*, 2004)

Juice. Juice is water plus some vitamins, minerals, and maybe some fiber. It's fine to start your day with a glass of juice, but remember that it adds a hefty dose of calories. Twelve ounces of orange juice, for example, gives you 168 calories—about what you'd get from three chocolate chip cookies. That's a high caloric price to pay for quenching your thirst. And again, the problem with drinking fruit juice instead of water is that many people don't compensate for the added calories by eating less. Most vegetable juices, by the way, have fewer calories than fruit juices, but check the label for both calories and salt before buying.

> ▶ *Dilution solution.* Try cutting your juice with a little water, gradually increasing the dilution over time till you're drinking one part juice to three parts water.

Much of what is sold as juice is really little more than fruit-flavored sugar water. Some "juice drinks" are obvious impostors, but others are harder to spot if you're only looking at the name and the package. Check the ingredient statement, though, and you'll see the difference immediately. Juice drinks—even those marketed as "juice" (often with fine-print qualifiers such as "drink" or "cocktail" in their names)—list water as the first ingredient, usually followed by high-fructose corn syrup and/or juice. Manufacturers put these drinks in splashy packaging with cues that say "fresh" and "light," hoping you'll reach for them as a healthy soft-drink alternative. But what you're getting is lots of empty calories—and a beverage that's nutritionally about the same as a soda.

Milk. An eight-ounce glass of whole milk contains 5 grams of saturated fat.

Drinking three glasses of it a day would be the saturated fat equivalent of eating twelve strips of bacon or a Big Mac with fries. Those three glasses would also add 450 calories to your diet, and the same amount of low-fat milk would still add 330 calories. *We don't recommend milk as a daily beverage for adults.* If you're concerned about calcium, getting it from a calcium/vitamin D supplement is a better bet (see Chapter 7).

Coffee. Good news, java-lovers. Despite centuries of suspicion and misinformation about the evils of coffee, it turns out to be a remarkably safe beverage. Yes, caffeine is a drug, and like any drug, if abused, it can become addictive. Yes, people who become dependent on it may get nasty headaches if they miss their morning cup. But in moderation, coffee is low on the list of foods that pose health risks, and may even have some beneficial effects. Moderate coffee drinkers tend to see a lower risk of developing kidney stones, gallstones, and type 2 diabetes. And coffee's antidepressant qualities are real and not insignificant. Suicide rates have been shown to be as much as 70 percent lower among coffee-drinkers as compared to non–coffee drinkers. The bottom line: *Drinking a few cups of coffee a day in the context of a healthy diet and activity level doesn't pose any health risks you need to worry about.* (Keep in mind that we mean regular cups of coffee with modest amounts of low-fat milk and/or sweetener—and not serial lattés or highly sweetened variations on milky themes.)

In fact, drinking up to six cups per day of filtered coffee seems to have little adverse effect, except for the jitters and insomnia experienced by some people (who don't often make the link between their coffee and these symptoms). A few studies have suggested a possible increase in fracture risk with four or more cups per day, but the findings are not consistent.

THE COFFEE-CHOLESTEROL CONNECTION

FILTERING COFFEE REMOVES substances that raise blood cholesterol levels; conversely, unfiltered coffee, which includes espresso and French press, can increase your cholesterol by a few points. So limiting intake of *unfiltered* coffee to one or two cups per day would be prudent unless your cholesterol level is really low.

Tea. Black tea and green tea come from the same plant. The difference is in how they're treated. Black tea is made by fermenting and drying the leaves of the tea plant. Green tea is made by steaming and drying tea leaves, without fermenting them. Both green and black tea contain caffeine—though in lower amounts than coffee—and the benefits that have been ascribed to coffee also apply to tea, including its mild antidepressant effect and its ability to help lower the risk of kidney stones and gallstones. There's been a lot of speculation about green tea helping to prevent cancer. It has been suggested that flavonoids (a kind of phytonutrient also found in berries, apples, tomatoes, broccoli, carrots, and onions) in green tea may lower rates of some forms of cancer, but there's been little clear scientific evidence to support this. Tea in moderation is fine. If you're concerned about caffeine, decaffeinated and herbal teas are a good option—another way to get the water you need, with a bit of added flavor, warmth, and satisfaction. Note that *yerba maté,* an ingredient in some teas, contains caffeine.

Alcohol. In moderation, alcohol is probably good for most people, but not everyone. (See Chapter 6.)

Sports drinks. For strenuous exercise that lasts longer than an hour, sports drinks can be a good way to stay hydrated and fueled without stopping to eat. Sports drinks give you a quick hit of energy from glucose, and they restore electrolytes that can be lost with sustained vigorous activity. The glucose helps in the absorption of those electrolytes and also helps prevent hypoglycemia, which can occur after several hours of sustained hard exercise (the phenomenon athletes call "hitting the wall"). Drinks such as Gatorade don't actually hydrate better than water, but because they're flavored and sweet, you're likely to drink them more often than you would water. If that works for you, fine. But for typical exercise activities such as cycling or walking for 20 to 30 minutes, your carbohydrate stores will be adequate if you eat slowly digested carbohydrates with meals (see Chapter 3) before exercising, and then just make a conscious choice to drink more water. Another solution, if you're going to be exerting a lot of energy over a sustained period of time, is to drink diluted orange juice and munch on a few salty snacks. If your activity brings about continuous sweating, this is one of those rare times when taking some extra salt is a good idea.

Dr. Willett's Science Bites
Fighting Kidney Stones with Fluids

PASSING A KIDNEY stone can be one of the most painful experiences imaginable. If you're not interested in discovering this firsthand, stay hydrated. Drinking plenty of fluids to maintain a good flow of urine and avoid the buildup of sludge in the kidney has long been thought to be a wise preventive measure. In fact, in both the Nurses' Health Study and Health Professionals' Follow-up Study, participants who drank more fluids had a lower risk of kidney stones. Women who drank more than ten glasses of fluids a day had a 40 percent lower risk than those who drank fewer than six glasses a day. Interestingly, *coffee, tea, and alcoholic beverages seem to be particularly beneficial for kidney stone prevention,* perhaps because they have a flushing effect. Consumption of grapefruit juice, which is known to have unusual metabolic effects, was related to a higher risk. (Source: Curhan, G., *Annals of Internal Medicine,* 1998, and Curhan, G., *American Journal of Epidemiology,* 1996)

IT'S IMPORTANT TO acknowledge that some sodium is necessary for our health, to maintain the proper distribution of fluids inside and outside cells. If we run low, from heavy sweating on a hot day during strenuous exercise, for example, and don't replace the sodium, our blood volume goes down, our blood pressure falls, we get weak, and we become mentally disoriented. If this situation weren't corrected and became extreme, it could even cause death. Sodium is important stuff, and that's why we have a taste for salt. For most of us, though, insufficient sodium is not something to worry about. Most people get far more than they need—often from unexpected sources, such as a bowl of commercial breakfast cereal or a serving of cottage cheese. A gram (that is, 1,000 milligrams, if you're not mathematically inclined) of sodium per day is plenty for the average person. Yet most of us in the United States take in much more. Average sodium consumption in the United States is more like 3,000 to 5,000 milligrams of sodium. That adds up to nearly two teaspoons of salt per day. Such a highly salty diet does tend to raise blood pressure, and thus our risk of heart attack and stroke, and has no positive function for anyone. The best approach is to slowly reduce the amount of salt we use to prepare food; in doing so we don't really miss it. Processed foods are the main stealth sources for sodium, so do read labels carefully. The current dietary reference intake (DRI) for sodium on food labels is 2,400 milligrams per day, but it is better to aim for less.

The How of H_2O

When it comes to hydration, the best advice we can offer you is this: *Stay hydrated, and make water your liquid of choice.* If you like, include coffee or tea in the mix. A bit of juice is okay, but generally speaking, make the shift toward more water. The *hydr-* in "hydration" comes from the Greek word for water. Take that as a hint. It's simply the best hydrator you can drink.

- ▶ *Six glasses a day.* Drink a glass of water between each meal and one with each meal. Six glasses of water a day, plus a diet like *Eat, Drink, and Weigh Less* that includes plenty of vegetables and fruits, will keep you where you need to be.
- ▶ *Drink before you eat.* Take the edge off your appetite by drinking a glass or two of water—or a cup of hot vegetable broth (page 171) a few minutes before you eat. You'll feel fuller and you'll be likely to eat less.
- ▶ *Water with meals, but . . .* The one drawback to "washing your food down" with any liquid is that it can cause you to chew less, and chewing is an important part of breaking down your food for optimal

digestion and absorption of nutrients—especially when you're eating a lot of whole grains, legumes, vegetables, fruits, and other fibrous foods. So be conscious of how and when you sip and chew.

▶ *Move beyond aquatic apathy.* Sure, tap water can be boring (and even revolting, if it's highly chlorinated). If you have trouble motivating yourself—or even *remembering*—to drink more of it, you're not alone. But make just about any conscious change in the way to think about, buy, serve, and drink water, and you'll be prompted to drink more of it. Here are some suggestions:

- *Treat yourself to bottled water.* Of course, it's more expensive than the "free" stuff that comes out of the tap, and in many communities, tap water tastes just as good. But manufacturers have created a whole industry around the psychological power of the bottle, and you can tap into that power, too. Keep small bottles of water in the fridge and "treat yourself" to them when you get the urge for a more caloric drink.

- *Buy a water filter pitcher.* Again, the effect is as much psychological as physiological. Regardless of what impurities that filter may be removing, the act of consciously filling the pitcher and putting it in the refrigerator keeps "water on the brain," reminding you to drink it more often.

- *Add sparkle.* Sparkling water—whether it's expensive imported mineral water or supermarket-brand club soda—is water. But it's got that extra something that many people find gratifying. If that's you, give yourself permission to buy it by the case and keep a few bottles in your refrigerator at all times. Try it a few times and it will become a habit—one that's worth every penny it costs if it means you get the water you need. And sparkling water has the added benefit that it makes some people feel a bit more full than still water, thus helping them to eat less.

- *Put it on ice.* Simple, yet effective. Take a few extra seconds to scare up some ice cubes. They'll make that glass of water more refreshing and pleasant to drink—and thus, less likely to languish on your desk or dinner table.

- *Flavor your water.* If even bottled water still feels boring and easy to forget, add a little flavor. Add a few slices of lemon, lime, or orange, or a splash of fruit juice to still or sparkling water to give it a little lift.

- *Tea up.* Keep a pitcher of iced herbal tea in the refrigerator to drink throughout the day. Get in the habit of brewing a cup of herbal tea to go along with between-meal snacks.

Water Regularly for Best Results

The principle here is straightforward: Drink plenty of liquids and avoid drinking empty calories. And for most of us, the easiest way to put that principle into practice is simply to make the shift from soda, juice, and other soft drinks to the clear, refreshing benefits of water.

6

Drink Alcohol
in Moderation (Optional)

A TOAST TO YOUR HEALTH

A GLASS OF WINE at the end of a long day helps melt away stress and heightens the pleasure of a meal. And the good news is, for most people, *wine—or any alcohol in moderation—can actually be beneficial to health.*

You've no doubt heard about the "French paradox"—the unexpectedly low rate of heart disease in France, despite a diet famous for its fatty foods. Researchers pointed to the red wine in the diet as the explanation. Yes and no. It's a combination of that, and the overall lifestyle and diet in parts of France, especially in the South, where the style of eating is more typically Mediterranean.

But there is more than a drop of truth to the red wine theory. Studies have shown that moderate consumption of alcohol—and not just red wine, but white wine, spirits, beer, and any beverage containing alcohol, does protect against heart disease and ischemic strokes, and there is increasing evidence suggesting that it also protects against diabetes, gallstones, and kidney cancer. Drinking alcohol raises levels of HDL (good) cholesterol and reduces the formation of arterial blood clots, which can cause heart attacks.

A Drink a Day Can Keep Heart Attacks at Bay

DOZENS OF STUDIES have shown that the risk of heart attacks in men and women who consume moderate amounts of alcohol is 30 to 40 percent lower than in those who do not drink. But some have claimed that the *type* of alcoholic beverage is important, with red wine being particularly beneficial because of the antioxidants it contains. Whether the pattern of drinking makes a difference has also been debated. To examine these issues, we studied the relation of alcohol consumption to risk of heart attack in more than 38,000 healthy men. During twelve years of follow-up, 1,418 men experienced a heart attack. *We found a 30 to 40 percent lower heart attack risk among men who consumed alcohol on most days of the week. But we also found that consuming a similar total amount concentrated in one or two days was not beneficial.* Whether the alcoholic beverage was consumed with meals or at other times did not appear to matter. Also, the benefits were not limited to any specific type of alcoholic beverage; in particular, *consumption of red wine did not confer greater reductions in risk for the same amount of alcohol.* (Source: Mukamal, K., *New England Journal of Medicine,* 2003)

So What Does "Moderate" Mean?

Men who have one or two alcoholic drinks a day are 30 to 40 percent less likely to have heart attacks than men who don't drink alcohol. The same benefits apply to women, though studies have also shown that one to two drinks a day can increase the risk of developing breast cancer. This is particularly true for women who don't get enough of the B vitamin known as folic acid in their diets. The same applies to colon cancer for both men and women—the increased risk with alcohol consumption seems to occur mainly among people whose diet is low in folic acid. So taking a multivitamin that contains folic acid is particularly important for people who drink alcohol.

Quantifying "moderation" is tricky, because so many factors come into play. But as a general guideline for healthy adults with no family history of alcoholism, *moderation means up to two drinks a day for men and one for women and older people.* (Women appear to metabolize alcohol less rapidly, and are, on average, smaller.)

As far as lowering the risk of heart disease is concerned, the benefits of consuming moderate amounts of alcohol appear to be consistent whether it is consumed with food or not. But establishing a pattern of drinking alcohol primarily with meals may help encourage moderation in general.

The Dark Side

Alcohol does, of course, present risks. It is addictive, especially in people who have a family history of alcoholism. It's the cause of about a third of traffic fatalities. And excessive drinking is a major cause of preventable deaths from liver disease, a variety of cancers, high blood pressure, and a progressive weakening of the heart and other muscles. Even at moderate levels, alcohol impairs judgment and slows reaction time. It can disrupt healthy sleep. And it interacts in potentially dangerous ways with a variety of medications, including acetaminophen (i.e., Tylenol), antidepressants, and other drugs.

Alcohol offers little benefit and adds potential risk to pregnant women and their unborn children, and to people with liver disease. For anyone under forty, its health benefits are negligible because the risk of heart disease is low at that age.

The Upside

But despite all that, alcohol in moderation can be helpful. If you're a man with no history of alcoholism who is at moderate to high risk for heart disease, a daily alcoholic drink will reduce that risk. If you are a woman with no history of alcoholism, remember that even a drink a day can increase your risk of breast cancer, but keep in mind, also, that a daily supplement of folic acid (as part of a multivitamin supplement) appears to prevent that increased risk. And if you're someone who can't seem to raise their HDL cholesterol level to where it should be despite a healthy diet and exercise, a drink or two a day may be particularly beneficial.

If you already drink alcohol, do keep it moderate. If you don't, don't feel you need to start. You can get similar benefits just by beginning to exercise or by upping the intensity and duration of your exercise program. No book can give you definitive answers about how much alcohol is right for you. As with all important diet and lifestyle decisions, it's a good idea to talk to your health-care provider about how your personal history and health concerns fit into the picture. Cheers!

Take a Multivitamin
Every Day

MULTIVITAMINS: GOOD, CHEAP HEALTH INSURANCE

FOR ABOUT A dime a day, you can enjoy the benefits of some pretty decent health insurance. It comes in pill form—as a multivitamin.

Vitamins used to be thought of as nutrients needed in small amounts to prevent diseases like scurvy and rickets. As those diseases became less common, people generally paid less attention to vitamins. But all that has changed in recent years as more and more research has pointed to the power of the vitamins and other nutrients found in a standard multivitamin to prevent heart disease, cancer, osteoporosis, and other chronic diseases.

An Addition, Not a Replacement

Taking a vitamin supplement is, of course, not a replacement for healthy eating. As we discussed in Chapter 1, no pill could give you the vast array of healthful nutrients and natural chemicals found in foods—or the combinations of those nutrients that work in synergy to keep you healthy. But a vitamin supplement can be a reliable backup plan—a way to fill any nutrient gaps that can show up from time to time, even in a healthy diet.

Folic acid, and vitamins B$_6$, B$_{12}$, D, and E are the five vitamins most people don't get enough of from their diets. Even the 21-Day Diet outlined in Chapter 12 can't guarantee that you'll get enough of them. Eating more fruits and vegetables, wonderful and healthful though they may be, won't give you much vitamin D, for example. And adding more whole grains doesn't gain you much vitamin B$_6$. If you drink alcohol, as we discuss in Chapter 6, you should take some additional folic acid. In short, taking a multivitamin is a safe, easy, inexpensive way to *complement* healthy eating.

What Kind Should You Buy?

Some multivitamins also include minerals. If you follow the healthy eating guidelines outlined in the *Eat, Drink, and Weigh Less* program, you probably won't need to buy a supplement with minerals, because you're likely to get enough of them from your food. Of course, if you want that extra safety net, it's fine. For menstruating women, especially those who don't eat much red meat, we recommend a vitamin supplement with minerals that include iron, which will help replace iron lost in menstruation.

Don't be taken in by fancy labels and promises of "megadoses" or "all natural" sources. Any RDA-level multivitamin—including a store brand—will give you most of what you need. One exception is likely to be vitamin D; the RDA is only 400 international units (IU) per day, but recent studies show that most people would be better off with at least 1,000 IU per day. At the moment, only a few multivitamins include this amount, but we hope more will do so soon.

Dr. Willett's Science Bites
Multivitamins Can Reduce Colon Cancer Risk

SEVERAL STUDIES IN animals and humans have shown that risk of colon tumors can be reduced by higher intakes of vitamin D or folic acid, one of the B vitamins. Because multivitamins are an important source of these nutrients, we examined the use of these supplements in relation to the risk of colon cancer among more than 88,000 women in the Nurses' Health Study. During fourteen years of follow-up, 442 women developed colon cancer. We saw little evidence of benefit for less than ten years of multivitamin use, but *after ten or more years, the risk of colon cancer appeared to be reduced by more than half as compared to the risk among women who did not use multivitamins.* With further follow-up of this group, we found that the benefit appeared to be greater among women who consumed alcohol (which increases the need for folic acid) and among those with a parent or sibling who had been diagnosed with colon cancer. (Source: Giovannucci, E., *Annals of Internal Medicine*, 1998)

Multivitamins Can Prevent Birth Defects

SEVERAL DECADES AGO, a British physician noted that major birth defects of the brain and spinal cord (spina bifida and anencephaly) occurred more frequently to mothers with poor diets, and additional studies found that rates of these defects were lower in mothers who took multivitamins. To test this directly, researchers in the United Kingdom randomly assigned women at high risk for these birth defects to take multivitamins containing folic acid, multivitamins without folic acid, or a placebo. Those who received multivitamins containing folic acid had a 72 percent lower risk of having a child affected by these birth defects as compared with the other groups. Subsequent studies showed that this benefit was also seen in women who did not have a high risk for birth defects. Based on this evidence, *it is now recommended by the Centers for Disease Control and other professional groups that all women of reproductive age who might possibly become pregnant take a multivitamin containing folic acid (which would be almost any standard multivitamin)*. Once a pregnancy has been diagnosed, it is usually too late to start, because these defects occur about four weeks after the embryo begins to develop. (Source: MRC Vitamin Study Research Group, *Lancet*, 2000)

Consider Vitamin E While You're at It

Several large studies among patients with heart disease have shown that separate supplements of vitamin E that contain amounts well above the RDA are not beneficial and therefore not recommended. The jury is still out on the use of vitamin E for people without existing heart disease. In a recent study among healthy women, those who took vitamin E supplements had only a 10 percent lower risk of heart attacks than did those who took a placebo, and this did not prove statistically significant. There was, however, a 24 percent lower risk of dying from all forms of cardiovascular disease combined, which would be an important benefit.

The amount of vitamin E present in food or in multivitamins isn't enough to reach the levels that may reduce cardiovascular disease, that is, 400 to 800 IU per day. Until further evidence is available, we suggest an extra vitamin E supplement for most men and post-menopausal women without existing heart disease, which means a separate pill, taken when you take your multivitamin. Because vitamin E can reduce the blood's ability to clot, people on blood-thinners should consult their health-care providers before taking vitamin E supplements.

Calcium—If You Need It, Get It from a Supplement

No one really knows how much calcium an adult needs each day, but the current recommended daily intakes of more than 1,000 milligrams are probably higher than necessary. An intake of 500 milligrams is probably enough, and the current English recommendation of 700 milligrams per day is likely to prove more than sufficient. If you feel you need to get more, keep in mind that a high consumption of dairy products is probably not the best source. Supplements are a better way to go, because they have no calories and saturated fat, and they're far more convenient and less expensive than several servings of dairy products. If you do buy a calcium supplement, get a calcium plus vitamin D combination; the extra vitamin D is likely to fill a gap in your nutrient stores. Also, there is powerful evidence showing that weight-bearing activities such as brisk walking—and weight-training, for upper body bones—greatly reduce risk of fractures associated with osteoporosis. The bottom line: If you want to prevent bone fractures, forget the milk and take your cow for a walk.

A Daily Habit

Make a multivitamin part of your daily diet. Buy a compartmentalized pill reminder box and stock it with multivitamins and whatever other daily supplements you choose to take. Or set a nice-looking pillbox on the table and refill it on the same day every week. You can take supplements before, after, or during a meal, but establish a routine so you don't forget altogether. We recommend drinking a glass of water before every meal (see Chapter 5), and that habit can dovetail nicely with this one.

8

Move
More

EXERCISE: START WITH THIRTY MINUTES A DAY

S O FAR, WE'VE talked about what to eat and drink and what not to—the intake side of the equation. But physical activity—the output side—is just as important. Exercise is about more than simply burning off fuel. We tend to oversimplify the equation, putting food on one side and deprivation and exercise on the other side. It's like a balance sheet that tells us, "You ate that cheese Danish. Now you'd better skip lunch, hit the gym, and burn it off." No pain, no gain, right? Well, not exactly.

We want you to think about this balance sheet in a different way. First of all, physical activity never needs to be "pain." Second, while it does burn calories, it's not a way to compensate for overindulging in empty calories. Third, it can be a hugely, undeniably, delightfully important part of living well and enjoying good health. Other than not smoking, weight control is the single best thing you can do to get healthy and stay healthy. And physical activity is not only an essential part of weight control, it can also offer a host of other health benefits.

As balance sheets go, this one may sound strange, but it's true nonetheless: Both sides are *positives*. You can eat well and deliciously, *and* you can derive the benefits of both weight maintenance and a longer, healthier life by making enjoyable, regular physical activity a part of your life.

Physical activity can help protect you from developing heart disease, high blood pressure, and high cholesterol. It can help defend you from certain cancers—including colon and breast cancer—as well as adult-onset diabetes, arthritis, and osteoporosis. It can also help improve your digestion, prevent constipation, lift your mood, clarify your thinking, relieve symptoms of depression, and improve your self-image. As feelings of well-being are stimulated through oxygenation and movement, cravings often subside, and in the process, choices about "indulgence food" can become less loaded and easier to deal with. And yes, on top of all that, physical activity helps you control your weight.

Exercise, Fat, and Muscle—the Total Picture

Exercise burns calories that would otherwise be stored by your body as fat. It also builds muscles. You knew that. But did you know that building muscle, or at least maintaining it, is an essential part of weight control?

Your muscles burn calories constantly—even when you're sleeping. They burn more, of course, when you engage in physical activity. But what's just as important is that physical activity also stimulates muscle cells to grow and divide. *Build more muscle and your body uses more energy, even at rest.*

If, on the other hand, you're very sedentary, your muscles will gradually shrink. You'll burn fewer calories at rest, and, to make matters worse, lost muscle is usually replaced by fat. Before long, you're caught in a vicious cycle. The more the balance shifts from muscle to fat, the more your metabolism slows down. That means you need less energy, so more of the food you eat goes into your body's fat stores instead of being used as fuel.

The more your fat-to-muscle ratio tips toward fat, *the easier it becomes to gain weight and the harder it becomes to lose it.* And the extra weight you gain makes it more difficult—and less appealing—to exercise, so your metabolism slows even further. You increase your risk of diabetes, heart disease, and stroke, and these risks may not always be fully reversible, even with weight loss. In other words, it's never too soon to start exercising regularly.

Remember, too, that when it comes to fat and muscle, the bathroom scale can't tell you the whole story. For an inactive person, a weight gain of 10 pounds over a few years might actually be a gain of 15 pounds of fat and a *loss* of 5 pounds of muscle. That's the balance shift you need to get control of, and the best way to do that is simply to get enough exercise.

How Much Is Enough?

Start with thirty minutes a day. Just about any kind of activity that gets your whole body moving will do the trick. Studies have shown that brisk walking offers many of the same benefits as more vigorous exercises, such as jogging. The more intense the exercise, of course, the more calories you'll burn. Activities like running or working out on an elliptical training machine give you a cardiovascular workout in a shorter time than lower-intensity activities such as walking.

But the good news is that you can get the workout you need, starting right now, just by *moving around* for thirty minutes a day—and those active minutes don't even have to be all in one stretch. However, we suggest working toward finding thirty minutes of time for physical activity, because it's the easiest way to be sure you're really getting the exercise you need. But if that's not realistic for you, at least at first, break it into manageable chunks.

Start by assessing your "exercise personality." Do you love solitude and long for more time just to gather your thoughts? Do you enjoy the motivation and social interaction that comes from working out with other people? Do you get a kick out of competing—or are you more interested in beating your own personal best? Pick realistic, enjoyable forms of physical activity that fit your personal style.

- ▶ *Walk the walk.* If you've got the time, walk briskly for thirty minutes or more a day. This can be as simple as finding ways to add more walking to your day. Get off the bus or train one or two stops early and walk the rest of the way. Park a little farther away. Walk around the block at lunchtime. Take the stairs instead of the elevator. (Remember, walking *down* a set of stairs is also exercise; it builds balance and coordination, and, because it's weight-bearing, it's a good calcium-retention strategy.) It's all good, and it all adds up.
- ▶ *Beat boredom.* If walking isn't your idea of a good time, spice it up. Listen to music, the radio, or audiobooks. Or make regular dates to walk with friends and use the time to get caught up.
- ▶ *Choose human-powered alternatives.* Go for the broom instead of the vacuum; the rake or shovel instead of the leaf- or snow-blower; your bike instead of the car.
- ▶ *Boogie to the beat.* Put a CD player in your kitchen so you can move and groove to the music as you cook or clean. Turn on the tunes in your living room and just dance (especially when no one else is around).
- ▶ *Buy a punching bag.* Jab away excess stress and get your workout at the same time. Treat yourself to a pair of boxing gloves while you're at it.
- ▶ *Low-tech is okay.* Besides rowing machines and Stair Masters (which, if you have them, you use, right?), simpler home equipment can include a chin-up bar placed strategically in a doorway you pass through often, a jump rope, or a small, portable trampoline that can be stored in a closet. (Take it out of the closet and jump your way through your favorite radio program on a rainy Saturday!)

- *Learn a new sport.* Pick one you've always wanted to try. Whether it's tennis, swimming, ballet, or jai alai, what matters is that you move and that you have fun.
- *Make the most of prime time.* When you watch TV, instead of sitting on the couch munching, sit on the floor, stretching—and doing a few sit-ups and push-ups during the commercials. Even better, put a stationary bike or other exercise machine in front of the TV and work out as you watch.
- *Move through the day.* Get up and walk around during work breaks. If you live in a house with stairs, go up and down while talking on the phone. Just plain fidget more. It all adds up!
- *Make it a class act.* If you're a "joiner," and you like social interaction, find a dance or exercise class—you'll work out and expand your social network at the same time.

Dr. Willett's Science Bites
Physical Activity—Does the Type Matter?

THE BENEFITS OF physical activity in reducing risk of heart disease have now been documented in dozens of long-term studies, but the role of specific forms of activity has been less clear. To examine this issue in detail, we followed more than 44,000 men in the Health Professional's Follow-up Study for twelve years, during which 1,700 participants experienced a heart attack. After adjusting for smoking, diet, and other risk factors, *the most active men had a 30 percent lower risk of heart disease than the most sedentary. Those engaging in more intense levels of activity had the lowest risk.* For example, men who ran for more than an hour per week had a 42 percent lower risk as compared with men who did not run, and brisk walking for thirty minutes or more per day was associated with an 18 percent lower risk. Also, men who trained with weights for thirty or more minutes per week had a 23 percent lower risk than those who did not use weights. *Almost any form of physical activity will be beneficial, but these findings indicate that higher intensity forms of activity provide additional benefit for reducing risk of heart disease. And resistance exercises, even for five minutes per day, can also contribute to lower risks.* (Source: Tanasescy, M., *Journal of the American Medical Association*, 2002)

PEDAL POWER

BY BIKING TO work, Walter gets thirty minutes of enjoyable, head-clearing exercise every day. It's actually faster than driving and parking, saves the expense of

(continued on next page)

owning a second car (not to mention the parking fees and gas), and reduces air pollution and global warming. Biking may not be for everyone, but for Walter and his wife, commuting by bike was an important factor in deciding where to live. (A note to cycling enthusiasts: As bicycles have evolved, they've become so efficient that many people get little workout from a typical, flat, cross-town ride. The trick is to ride a bit faster or include a few hills in your route.)

Resistance—and Why You Need It

What we've described so far is mostly aerobic activity (the kind that makes your heart and lungs work faster). But there's another kind of exercise you also need: *resistance training*. This kind of exercise involves working specific muscle groups to *lift or push weight*. It can take the form of old-fashioned no-equipment exercise that uses your body as the weight (e.g., push-ups, pull-ups, sit-ups); working out with weights or exercise equipment; or training with elastic exercise bands.

Resistance exercise becomes more important after the age of thirty because our muscles start to shrink due to declining levels of hormones such as estrogens and testosterone. The only way to counteract this shrinkage is to give the muscles more of a workout. It's important to remember that *each part of the body needs its own workout to maintain its muscles.*

Most of us work our legs by walking and climbing stairs, so the kind of activities we've described above will provide both aerobic exercise and some muscle-building for the legs. But our torsos, arms, and necks also need working out. The net effect of working all of our major muscle groups is significant. It will keep the muscles from shrinking; maintain strength that reduces the risk of falling as we get older; make our bones stronger because they respond to the muscles pulling on them; burn calories 24/7; reduce insulin resistance and thus the risk of diabetes; and make us look and feel better.

And for all its benefits, resistance training requires very little time. Even one or two minutes for each muscle group (ten to fifteen minutes total), three times a week can make a huge difference. Anyone can do resistance training, even people with serious heart disease or diabetes—though if you are over forty or have an existing disease, you should consult with your health-care provider before beginning.

No matter what your starting level, *begin gently and build up slowly over many weeks*; you will be amazed at what you can do after six months. If you are not familiar with this kind of exercise, a few sessions with a personal trainer are a worthwhile investment. A trainer can help you get started on the right track and steer you away from bad habits, so you get the maximum benefit from each exercise. Once you get going, you will become your own best expert about what works for your body and your schedule.

Do Whatever Moves You

You're inundated with images and information about exercise and fitness. But don't let anyone tell you how or what you have to do. It's not necessarily about joining a gym or training for a triathlon—unless, of course, you want to. *Just aim toward moving thirty minutes a day.* Find a way to do it that clicks with you. Start slow, but start—and stick with it. Let it quietly become a habit. Before long, instead of having to *find* time for exercise, you'll want to *make* time for it. And when it comes to investing in your long-term health, that will be time well spent.

9

Eat Mindfully All Day Long

A GUIDE TO DIETARY CONSCIOUSNESS-RAISING

ALONG WITH EXERCISE, being truly conscious of the food choices you make is the key to a healthy diet and to achieving and maintaining a healthy weight. And, although most diet books focus on the question of *what* you eat, we want you to understand that *how* you eat is just as important.

It comes down to two basic ideas: *pace* and *mindfulness*. *Pace* means deliberately eating enough at regular intervals so that you have the fuel you need to function well and keep your blood sugar at a relatively consistent level. *Mindfulness* means paying attention to your food choices—and savoring every bite, instead of nibbling, inhaling your food without chewing enough, or just plain eating without much thought. What we want you to avoid is mindless "sleep-eating." Here's why.

Understanding Hunger

You're hungry—or at least you think you are. You reach for food. What could be more straightforward? But, too often, we misunderstand hunger. We think, "I'm not really hungry right now. I'll skip breakfast." Or, "I'm starving! I need a snack." Or, "I'm bored (or lonely or frustrated or anxious). Let me eat cake!" All of these impulses seem perfectly natural and appropriate.

But often what we're experiencing is hunger of a sort that food can't stave off. And when we eat to satisfy this kind of psychological hunger, we tend to eat very quickly—maybe even without breathing. A good first step when you feel this kind of emptiness approaching is to identify its true nature.

True physiological hunger means you're running out of stored fuel. Your blood-sugar level drops and your brain starts waving red flags like crazy. It's distracting and unpleasant. You lose your ability to concentrate and you get grouchy and spaced out. So you reach for the nearest food, often instinctively grabbing something with sugar or easily digested carbohydrates, the stuff your body and brain know is the fastest ticket to getting your blood sugar back up.

As we discussed in Chapter 3, this sets off a cycle of eating (and often overeating) followed immediately by a spike in blood sugar. What follows, in turn, is a responsive surge of insulin production, which can drive blood sugar too low and start the whole process over again. This pattern is unhealthy in the long term, and in the medium-to-short term it's not a good way to manage food for optimal energy and weight control.

The way to stay out of this loop is to *remove hunger from the equation as much as you can.* Eat three good meals a day, stay hydrated, and snack smartly in between if necessary, and you should seldom feel debilitating hunger. (A little edge of appetite, on the other hand, won't hurt you, and is to be expected from time to time, especially if you are on a weight-loss plan.) Avoid ravenous hunger, and chances are you'll avoid misusing or misinterpreting hunger as a cue.

The Fallacy of Skipping Meals

How many times have you gotten to 2:30 P.M. without having had a chance to eat lunch? "Oh, well," you think. "I'm trying to lose weight. I need to take in fewer calories. And I'm going out for dinner. I'll just forgo lunch and eat this little bag of pretzels. And that won't really count because the pretzels are low-fat and, besides, snack calories are basically invisible when I've skipped lunch."

It happens. But try to avoid skipping meals. Not only does it send you off on that bumpy, peak-and-trough blood-sugar ride, but it can cause overeating later on, because you're so hungry. This makes skipping meals a possible contributor to weight gain. The best plan is to eat a nourishing breakfast, lunch, and dinner, and, if you need them, have healthy, modest, nutritionally significant snacks between meals.

Of course, it's completely natural to be a little hungry from time to time. And we're not saying you should stuff yourself all day so you're never hungry.

What we *are* saying is, *don't let yourself get too hungry.* What you're going for is a feeling of *satiety*—neither uncomfortably full nor running on empty, but the sweet spot in between. The opposite of satiety, in dietary terms, is deprivation—the mopey feeling that you're missing out on all the fun, and the reason even the best-intentioned dieters often fail to stick with the program. Don't starve yourself. Stay comfortably sated with healthy food. Your feelings of deprivation will be far less frequent and intense, and your positive attitude will shore you up and keep you going.

And remember, when hunger does hit you, it's helpful to ask why. Chances are you skimped on a meal or skipped it altogether, or you're feeling an emotional need that's masquerading as a physical one. Or maybe you're actually thirsty. Whatever the cause, when you're tempted to reach for food to make yourself feel better, don't go on auto pilot and head for the kitchen. Take a moment. Take a deep breath. Get a glass of water. Take another deep breath. Close your eyes and clear your mind. Wait ten or fifteen minutes. Then, if you're still feeling hungry, eat something sensible.

It All Begins with Breakfast

When it comes to smoothing out the peaks and troughs of hunger all day long, a good breakfast starts things off on exactly the right track. Skip breakfast, or make less-than-optimal food choices, and it's easy to set off a chain of overeating that lasts till bedtime.

It's called "breakfast" for a reason. When you wake up, your blood sugar is at "fasting level"—not a state in which you perform optimally for long. Breaking that fast powers you up for the day ahead, and how you choose to break it is important. Big farmhouse breakfasts once fueled people for manual labor with a hearty combination of eggs, meat, dairy, and carbohydrates. We may not be headed out for a day of work in the fields like our ancestors, but we still need sustaining, slow-burning fuel. Unfortunately, the typical modern-world breakfast options—at least the ones that are the most available, convenient, fast, and filling—are usually the nutritional opposite of that kind of farmhouse fare. They tend to be mostly highly refined carbohydrates (including most breakfast cereals, bagels, and breads) and foods with a lot of sugar (such as muffins, doughnuts, and pastries). In other words, our default breakfast choices lean toward foods that find their way quickly into the bloodstream and leave us feeling hungry sooner than they should.

Replace these foods with less quickly absorbed elements—such as good fat, some kind of fiber, a whole-grain food, or a good dose of protein—and the release of sugar into your bloodstream will slow down. You'll be less likely to have midmorning cravings and more likely to eat a sensible lunch, and your energy level and concentration will stay more consistent all day long.

So, don't skip breakfast, and do eat a good mix of slowly digested foods. If you're just not hungry when you wake up, wait a bit, but try to eat—and eat well—within a few hours after the alarm clock goes off. And if you need extra help, here's a simple tip: Finish dinner no later than 8:00 P.M. and don't eat anything afterward. Try this for a few days. You may turn out to be someone who likes breakfast after all.

Here are a few simple breakfast guidelines:

- ▶ *Make the most of your toast.* Use whole-grain bread, and add a little nut butter or olive oil.
- ▶ *Switch from juice to fruit.* A glass of orange juice has twice as many calories as an orange. Eat a piece of fruit for breakfast, or purée it into a smoothie (pages 182–184). And avoid sugared fruit drinks altogether.
- ▶ *Add whole grains.* Switch your cold cereal to one whose first ingredient is a whole grain. (See page 266 for some cereal guidelines.) Or, if you can't let go of your beloved cornflakes, add in a few spoonfuls of leftover cooked whole grains—they'll add texture and nuttiness without depriving you of your familiar wake-up ritual. Try a whole-grain hot cereal, such as steel-cut oats, or one made from partially processed grains, such as rolled oats.
- ▶ *Try to include some good-quality protein.* It might be a handful of nuts tossed into your cereal, an egg, some yogurt, a piece of smoked fish, even beans or tofu. Keeping an open mind about savory options for breakfast will help you add a bit of protein that can sustain you for hours.
- ▶ *Grab and go.* If you have a small appetite and/or need whatever you are eating to be portable (the "one hand on the breakfast, the other hand on the wheel" syndrome), or you need to eat at your desk, try one of our delicious, nutritionally dense Nuggets and Gems (pages 179–181). They travel well and stave off hunger for hours!

Snack Strategically

We say it all the time: "It's just a snack." It's as if to say that what really matters are meals, and snacks are just a bite or two that hardly warrant any real thought or attention. But as meals, life, and work blur into an increasingly undifferentiated whirl of food consumption, snacking often *is* eating. Replacing meals with snacks is not a good idea. And snacking deserves special attention. Again, it's not just what you snack on, it's how and why.

Feeling hungry between meals probably means that you didn't get enough quality nutrition at your last meal. Or perhaps you've been particularly active and you need fuel. But often, it's not so much a matter of fuel levels at all. Snacking—like all eating—can also be a response to boredom or stress. What's helpful in managing how you snack is to think about where your snacking urge is coming from, and then feed *that* need.

▶ *You may be thirsty.* Mild dehydration can make you feel hungry, even though what you really need is water. Drink a glass before you get a snack. And fight the temptation to hit the soda machine.

▶ *You've got "restless mouth syndrome."* You're not exactly hungry, you're just feeling fidgety or maybe a little bored. Instead of chips or other highly refined salty snacks, try to eat something nutrient-light that's low in calories but can give you a lot of satisfying chewing, such as:
   • Baby carrots or other raw vegetables, eaten plain or dipped in Tangy Black-Bean Dip (page 189) or Hummus (page 190)
   • Slices of apple
   • Air-popped popcorn or puffed cereal, eaten one morsel at a time (no fistfuls!)
   • A few low-sugar gummy bears. No kidding. They won't add up to much calorically, and they'll make your restless mouth smile.

▶ *You're having trouble concentrating.* Try something light and refreshing, like:
   • A crisp, cold apple, or other fresh seasonal fruit
   • A tall, icy glass of unsweetened (or lightly fruit-sweetened) citrus-laced sparkling water or iced tea, with a big wedge of lemon or lime and/or a sprig of fresh mint
   • A big glass of three parts sparkling or still water with one part juice, over ice
   • A cup of hot tea with a little sweetener, with or without a splash of milk
   • Half of a high-quality protein bar (see page 268), eaten slowly
   • Twelve chocolate chips, melted on your tongue one at a time
   • Ten unsalted almonds, eaten slowly (unsalted because salt tends to make you want to eat more)
   • A handful of cherry tomatoes, olives, and/or celery sticks

▶ *You're feeling exhausted.* Eat a nutrient-dense snack with meaningful calories, such as:
   • A hit of big-time, pure protein. Sometimes you need just that, plain and simple, to get you back into gear. Go for a chunk of baked tofu, a hard-boiled egg, or a few slices of cold chicken, lean roast beef, or turkey breast.

- A small piece (½ ounce) of cheese (that's the size of half a piece of string cheese)
- 1 serving small brown rice cracker with dabs of nut butter
- Wedges of red or yellow bell pepper dipped in Hummus (see page 190)
- Yogurt (see page 267)
- A smoothie (see pages 182–184 and 267)
- A glass of low-fat chocolate milk or vanilla soy milk
- The other half of the high-quality protein bar
- Baked Coated Nuts (see pages 177–178)
- Super Trail Mix (see pages 175–176)

We've given you some options for "strategic snacking." (We've even included a list of safe treats to cover your possible cravings—see page 109.) But we want to make it clear that if you eat good, balanced meals, you shouldn't really need to do much snacking. And if your goal is weight loss or maintaining healthy weight, snacking can get in your way, because it's not always easy to remember to cut down your calories at meals to compensate for between-meal snacks. To sum it up: Eat three good meals a day—like the ones in the 21-Day Diet—and if you still feel the need to snack, snack consciously and moderately, remembering to breathe and drink water, too.

Dr. Willett's Science Bites
Snacking vs. Meals

DAVID JENKINS, WHO originated the concept of the glycemic index, studied the effect of increasing the frequency of eating on cholesterol and carbohydrate metabolism. Keeping the number of calories per day constant, food was given to two groups of seven men as either three meals or seventeen snacks. After two weeks, the men were given the alternative meal pattern. While on the snacking diet, the men's LDL (bad) cholesterol was 14 percent lower and their average insulin level decreased by 28 percent. Thus, *spreading calories out over the day provides a better metabolic picture than concentrating the calories in three large meals*. But keep in mind that breaking eating up into many small snacks makes it harder to have a clear sense of total calories consumed. And by eating slowly digested foods (such as whole-grain pasta as compared to potatoes) at regular meals, we can gain similar benefits. (Source: Jenkins D., *New England Journal of Medicine*, 1989)

INSTEAD OF INGESTING your serving of Super Trail Mix (or whatever snack you choose) in one large handful, put it on a plate or napkin, and pick up one morsel at a time. Place it in your mouth while paying full attention—instead of concentrating on doing something else. Or take a few minutes to cut an apple into wedges and put them on a plate rather than grabbing the whole fruit and wolfing it down in a few big bites. You'll eat less quickly this way, and with greater pleasure—which will make for a more sustaining, satisfying snack. Whatever you choose to munch on—whether it's Super Trail Mix, nuts, air-popped popcorn, or pieces of whole-grain cereal—go slowly and stretch out the experience. You'll feel calmer and fuller sooner.

Fullness and Mindfulness

Making good food choices and getting to a healthy weight start with awareness. Just *thinking* about how you eat can *change* how you eat. That may sound obvious, but put it into practice, and you'll find things start to shift as you begin to understand your eating habits and as you start seeing patterns that you never even noticed. Here are a few simple ways to start. You know them all already, but we all need reminders.

- ▶ *Eat slowly.* You'll automatically eat less, because your brain will have more time to receive and send signals of fullness. When you eat quickly, you short-circuit those signals, and it's easy to overeat. Think of it this way: No one ever gorges or binges slowly. That pretty much says it all.
- ▶ *Drink water first.* Start every meal with a glass of water and a few deep breaths to shift gears into mindful eating mode.
- ▶ *Taste and savor every bite.* You'll feel more satisfied, and you'll chew more thoroughly, which will help you digest your food and get the most out of it nutritionally.
- ▶ *Breathe and smile.* It sounds hokey, but taking deep breaths and smiling between bites of food helps you feel relaxed, focused, and content.
- ▶ *Don't multitask.* Take time out to eat for eating's sake. Sit at the table. Don't work or read (unless, of course, you're reading this list!). Look at your food. Smell the aromas. Taste the flavors. Relish the textures.
- ▶ *Try not to talk with your mouth full.* Seriously. It's not just a matter of etiquette. Again, it's all about being as conscious of your food as you can be.

- *After every three bites, put down your fork.* Chew, swallow, savor, repeat.
- *Seek satisfaction and healthy opulence.* Cooking good food and serving it in a pleasing way takes a little more time, but it makes you feel more content—more like you've really *eaten* and less like you've just been fed.
- *Be selective.* Don't just eat whatever's served to you, whether at home, at someone's house, or at a restaurant.
- *Stop before you're stuffed.* Before you go for seconds or thirds, wait five to ten minutes and then ask yourself if you're still hungry. The idea, in the long run, is to get into the habit of eating until you're satisfied, but never until you're uncomfortably, "Thanksgiving-dinner" stuffed. Except maybe on Thanksgiving.
- *Most of all, love your food.* Don't make food the enemy. Honor it with love and respect. Appreciate it, and it will treat you well.

The Nine Turning Points outlined in these chapters give you the fundamentals of eating right for weight control and long-term health. If there's one principle they all share, it's this: *Accentuate the positive.* Better, not less. Tastier, not more boring. Satiety, not deprivation. In diet management, as in life, happiness counts for a lot. And mindfulness is next to happiness. Smell the roses—and the rosemary. Enjoy your food. And take pride and pleasure in knowing you're making positive choices based on sound, proven principles. Now, let's put those principles into a simple tool you can start using today: *Your Body Score.*

10

Your
Body Score

A NUMBER THAT CAN CHANGE YOUR LIFE

THE BODY SCORE is a simple, powerful tool to help you lose weight and stay healthy. It distills the Nine Turning Points of weight management and healthy eating into a single, motivating number that you can use to gauge your progress. Like the *Eat, Drink, and Weigh Less* program, your Body Score is about total health in addition to weight loss. It shows you how to *add* food, rather than simply subtracting, and prevents self-starvation, which might help you lose weight in the short run, but usually results in a yo-yo effect of losing and gaining.

Here's what it promises: *Raise your score and you'll lower your weight and improve your health over the course of your life.*

And here's how it works:

- ▶ **Set a benchmark.** Before you begin the 21-Day Diet or the Warm-Up Plan, go through the Body Score Card, answering the questions based on the previous few days to determine your starting Body Score.
- ▶ **Keep a journal.** Writing down what you eat can be a helpful way to become more conscious of your eating overall. It's

also invaluable—at least at first—in helping you measure your Body Score as accurately as possible.

▶ *Scoring.* Tally your points—0, 1, or 2—for each question and add them up to arrive at your Body Score.

▶ *Daily at first.* As you begin either the 21-Day Diet or the Warm-Up Plan, go through the Body Score Card at the end of every day. At the outset, your goal is to raise your score as much as you can every day.

▶ *Weekly later.* After a few weeks—and when you've reached your target weight and want to stay there—go through the Body Score Card at the end of the week, using a journal, if you need to, as a reminder.

▶ *What about calories?* Because we want you to focus more on the qualitative aspects of the food and lifestyle choices you make than on the quantitative ones, your Body Score is not directly related to calories. But bear in mind that the recommended caloric intake for weight loss is 1,500 to 1,600 calories a day, with regular exercise. To get a sense of what that looks and feels like in food terms, read through the 21-Day Diet. We have counted the calories for you, so if you simply follow our portion-size indications, you'll end up in the 1,500 to 1,600 calorie per day range. If you want to delve further into your own calorie counting, there are plenty of Web sites that make it easy, for example, www.nutritiondata.com.

Evaluating Your Score:

Shoot for a range of 25 to 50. If you're already at 25 or above, congratulations! You're doing well. Keep up the good work, and try to raise your score as much as you can. A score of 50 means you're doing all the right things. Remember:

▶ *The higher your score, the more weight you'll lose, and the better you'll feel as your health and state of mind improve!*

▶ This score is not a grade. It's not about judgment or failure. Think of it as a Scrabble game you're playing with yourself. Focus on getting the highest score you can.

▶ You don't need to dive into the deep end. Even if you're not ready to start the 21-Day Diet, doing whatever you can to raise your score will help you start losing weight and improving your health.

▶ It's not a test, it's a tool—the Body Score is a formula for healthy weight loss that reduces the wisdom of decades of research and science into a number you can manage.

▶ This is not a competition. Everyone is a winner. Enjoy the game.

THE BODY SCORE CARD

		# OF POINTS	YOUR SCORE
WHAT YOU EAT			
A-LIST VEGETABLES (page 27)			
	Fewer than 2 servings a day	0	
	2 servings a day	1	
	3 or more servings a day	2	
A-LIST FRUITS (page 30)			
	Fewer than 1 serving a day	0	
	1 serving a day	1	
	2 or more servings a day	2	
WHOLE GRAINS AND WHOLE-GRAIN PRODUCTS			
	Fewer than 5 servings a week	0	
	One serving a day	1	
	More than one serving a day	2	
GOOD FATS			
	Zero or hardly any	0	
	Olive oil and other healthy oils, nuts, flax, and/or avocado once a day or less	1	
	Olive oil and other healthy oils, nuts, flax, and/or avocado a few times a day	2	
QUALITY PROTEIN			
	All or most from fatty meat and full-fat dairy	0	
	All or most from lean meat, fish, poultry, eggs, low-fat dairy	1	
	About half from legumes, whole grains, nuts, and other vegetable sources (the rest from lean meat, fish, poultry, eggs, low-fat dairy)	2	
BONUS POINTS—For each additional serving of these (beyond your first 3 vegetables on any given day), add 1 point per serving, 2 points if prepared with olive oil			
	Cooked A-List green vegetables (½ cup serving) (see page 27)	1 or 2	
	Tomatoes, raw or cooked (½ cup serving)	1 or 2	
	Salad greens, especially deeply colored ones, such as romaine, spinach, or arugula (1 cup serving)	1 or 2	
HOW, WHEN, WHY, AND WHERE YOU EAT			
PACE			
	I tended to eat very quickly.	0	

		# OF POINTS	YOUR SCORE
	I managed to make my meals last for an average of 5 to 10 minutes.	1	
	I stretched most meals to at least 15 minutes.	2	
LOCATION AND MODE			
	I tended to eat while standing, walking around the house, driving, talking on the phone, or in front of a TV or computer.	0	
	I mostly ate while sitting and reading.	1	
	I ate while sitting and relaxing—alone, or with others.	2	
FOCUS			
	I didn't think about my food when eating it, and don't remember much about it.	0	
	I noticed and enjoyed some of what I ate and remember some of it.	1	
	I paid full attention each time I ate, tasting and enjoying my food, and remember it well.	2	
PURPOSE			
	I ate mostly because I felt bored, lonely, or sad.	0	
	I usually ate because it was mealtime.	1	
	I ate because it was mealtime and I was really looking forward to eating.	2	
MEALS			
	I skipped meals here and there.	0	
	I ate 3 meals each day, but they were of varying quality and not all of them were balanced.	1	
	I ate 3 balanced meals of top quality each day.	2	
BREAKFAST			
	I ate no breakfast to speak of (except perhaps a bagel or pastry on some days, with or without coffee).	0	
	I ate a few bites of something healthy on most days.	1	
	I ate a full, healthy breakfast every day.	2	
BETWEEN MEALS			
	I snacked indiscriminately and for no particular reason, and can't really say what I ate or how much.	0	
	I had a few healthy snacks and a few "empty" ones.	1	
	I snacked when hungry on items recommended in this book (Snack Strategically, pages 91–94, and That Thing You Crave, page 109).	2	

(continued on next page)

		# OF POINTS	YOUR SCORE
AFTER DINNER			
	I ingested major calories between dinner and bedtime.	0	
	I had a light, healthy snack or a glass of low-fat milk once in a while between dinner and bedtime.	1	
	I had nothing after dinner in anticipation of my good breakfast the next morning.	2	
FOOD-POSITIVITY			
	I didn't do any focused grocery shopping or cooking at all.	0	
	I spent a little time on focused shopping and did a little cooking.	1	
	I made a point to shop well, spending time in the produce department and other healthy food venues, and enjoyed several sessions of simple cooking.	2	
SELF-SABOTAGE			
	I tempted myself by having sweets, ice cream, and/or unhealthy snacks in the house—and I lost the bet.	0	
	I tempted myself by having sweets, ice cream, and/or unhealthy snacks in the house—and I won the bet.	1	
	I decided not to have sweets, ice cream, and/or unhealthy snacks on the premises at all and focused on other things.	2	
HEALTHY BODY HABITS			
AEROBIC EXERCISE			
	I didn't.	0	
	I did some decent moving around on most days.	1	
	I did sustained brisk movement (walking, jogging, cycling, aerobic machines, swimming, etc.) for at least 30 minutes, at least 4 days during the week.	2	
RESISTANCE EXERCISE			
	I resisted.	0	
	I did a few chin-ups, pull-ups, push-ups—or a little weight-lifting a few times here and there.	1	
	I did 5 minutes or more of chin-ups, pull-ups, push-ups, or weight-lifting at least 3 times during the week.	2	
WATER			
	I drank only a few sips once in a while.	0	
	I drank a few glasses on most days.	1	
	I drank at least six 8-ounce glasses every day.	2	

	# OF POINTS	YOUR SCORE
SLEEP AND RELAXATION		
I was generally sleep-deprived and couldn't seem to catch up or find time to rest.	0	
I slept fairly well most nights and found some additional time to relax some of the time.	1	
I slept as much as I needed and made additional time to relax regularly.	2	
MULTIVITAMIN		
None	0	
Some days	1	
Every day	2	
WEIGHT MONITORING		
I haven't weighed myself in recent memory and am afraid to look.	0	
I weigh myself at least once a day, sometimes more.	0	
I weigh myself at least several times a week, tending to get on a scale whenever I see one.	0	
I weigh myself on the same scale once a week— at the same time of day and in the same clothing.	2	
BONUS POINTS—*Add 2 points per day for each of these:*		
Add two extra points if you did at least 30 minutes of aerobic exercise more than four times per week (within reason; make sure your doctor approves!).		
Add two extra points if you did resistance exercise for at least five minutes more than three times per week.		
Add two extra points if you had 1 to 2 alcoholic drinks (not more) on at least three days per week. (Points count only if you are at least 40 years old and have no reason to avoid alcohol.)		
WHAT YOU DON'T EAT		
WHITE BREAD, WHITE RICE, POTATOES, OR POTATO PRODUCTS		
Subtract 2 points every time per day you eat a serving of white bread, white rice, potatoes, potato products, or processed snack food.		
SUGAR-SWEETENED BEVERAGES		
Subtract 2 points for every serving per day of a sugar-sweetened beverage.		
TOTAL—YOUR BODY SCORE		

2

The Plans

11

The Warm-Up Plan

I F YOU DO nothing else now or ever, this simple, nonstructured approach will still make a difference. These guidelines are for when you:

- ▶ would like to move toward a healthier diet without giving up what's comforting and familiar
- ▶ plan to go on the 21-Day Diet, but prefer to get prepared, so it's not a sudden change
- ▶ want to lighten up and maybe lose a few pounds over the long haul without undertaking something measured and prescriptive
- ▶ might be overwhelmed by anything more than just a few bullet points (Don't worry. There are only ten.)
- ▶ want to start doing *something* immediately

Remember, this plan is an optional introduction or alternative. If you're ready to go for it, you can turn right to the 21-Day Diet on page 107 and start there.

Copy this page and post it somewhere visible. Then do these basic things. After a week, you should start noticing positive changes in your mood and your body.

- ► Eat a good breakfast within three hours of getting up. Don't skip this meal!
- ► Eat nothing after dinner.
- ► Exercise or move for at least thirty minutes every day. (Moderate activity, such as walking, is fine.)
- ► *Add* at least two servings of "A-List" vegetables daily. (See page 27.)
- ► *Add* at least one serving of "A-List" fruit daily. (See page 30.)
- ► Limit your "white starch" carbohydrate intake to just one serving daily, if any. Try to make the rest (or all) of your carbs whole wheat, whole grain, etc.
- ► Allow yourself one small dessert every other day. Eat it slowly and enjoy!
- ► Try to drink at least six 8-ounce glasses of water a day.
- ► Have some protein at each meal.
- ► Your alcohol allowance: One serving per day of wine, beer, or a non-sweetened mixed beverage (optional).

Read through the Nine Turning Points, thinking about how they can fit into your life. You can keep eating the foods you are used to, but make room on your plate—and in your day—for incorporating as many of those recommendations as you can. Remember to keep tabs on your weight once a week, using the same scale, at the same time of day, and in the same clothes. And don't forget to take a deep breath, eat slowly, and pop that daily multivitamin!

12

The 21-Day
Diet

BEFORE YOU BEGIN

THE 21-DAY DIET is a fully-laid-out, three-week menu plan. You can follow it verbatim if you wish or you can use it as a template.

Each day's approximate total of 1,500 to 1,600 calories is broken down to about the same number of calories in each breakfast (about 350), lunch (around 400), snack (up to 250), and dinner (500 to 600). So the meals and snacks are interchangeable from one day to another. If you find that you really love several of the meals and want to repeat them, go ahead and swap out some of the ones that appeal to you less. If you prefer one of the breakfasts over the others, for example, and would be happy having it every day, go ahead and do so. Or if certain snacks work better for you than others, switch them around. And when you're in a snack-pinch, you can substitute a good-quality protein bar (page 268) and still be in the right ballpark. Make this diet your own!

Plan-Hopping

Not only can you mix and match meals, you can do the same with plans. For instance, you might need to switch over to the Portable Plan while traveling, but then return to the 21-Day Diet when you come home. You might want to extend the three weeks into six weeks (just repeat the cycle) or just fall back on the Warm-Up Plan for a while. Fit this into your life as best you can.

Unlimited Foods

Each day, certain items are designated "unlimited," so that if you are still hungry, you can keep eating *something*. These choices are mostly vegetables—raw or roasted—for tasty off the radar snacking. But do be careful not to stuff yourself to the brink. That's never a good idea.

The Fallback Meals

If you are too busy to cook a given meal from the 21-Day Diet, or you just want to eat more simply, here are two meals you can always use as a replacement for any lunch or dinner:

The "Regular Plate"
- ▶ 1 serving Protein-of-Choice (pages 201–210)
- ▶ 2 or more servings green vegetables (pages 227–232, 234, 236–237)
- ▶ 1 serving orange vegetables (pages 224–226)
- ▶ ½ cup cooked whole grains (pages 54–56)

The Main-Dish Salad
- ▶ A big bowlful (quantity unlimited) of salad greens and all sorts of vegetables
- ▶ 1 serving Protein-of-Choice (pages 201–210)—cut up and tossed into the salad or arranged on top
- ▶ ½ cup cooked whole grains (pages 54–56), sprinkled into the salad
- ▶ Olive oil and vinegar—or one of our salad dressings (pages 198–200)

Yes, Substitutions

If you have trouble finding the time to cook, you can substitute some of the quicker recipes for the more labor-intensive. (Look through the recipe section, beginning on page 145.) Many of the vegetable recipes are interchangeable. If certain fruits and vegetables on the list are out of season, you can substitute something similar or use a frozen version. (Unsweetened raspberries, blueberries, and blackberries freeze and defrost very well. And frozen spinach or chopped broccoli can be pureed beautifully into soup. See pages 168–169.)

Treats

The 21-Day Diet's approximate daily intake of 1,500 to 1,600 calories is on the low end for some people. This leaves room for a treat now and then and for many, an occasional treat can be a very good idea, psychologically! That's why we have built into these menus some standard favorites, such as crackers and tortilla chips. (Friends of ours who have experimented with certain popular diets describe wistfully how much they miss foods that crunch.)

If, in addition, you crave your beloved slice of bread, glass of wine, or dish (½ cup) of ice cream, you may add one of those three things per day, and you will still lose weight, only perhaps at a slower rate.

Or you can choose *one* item per day from That Thing You Crave (below) to keep you happy without falling off the rails. You can also add these only once or twice a week—or not at all. It's up to you. For some people, this is a slippery slope, but for others, this small allowance can make a huge difference in their quality of life!

Also, although coffee and tea are suggested at breakfast only, feel free to drink them throughout the day if you wish, as long as you don't shortchange your intake of water.

THAT THING YOU CRAVE

Ten Safe Treats—One a Day Is Okay

IF YOU'RE FEELING treat-deprived, here's your menu. None of these, in the measured amount, will bust your diet. So if you feel the need, select a maximum of one per day. Measure out the prescribed amount, put it on a plate or into a small plastic bag (if applicable), and put the rest away at least until tomorrow.

- 2 sugar-free Fudgsicles
- 2 frozen unsweetened fruit juice bars
- 7 medium-size pretzels or 1 handful of "good" (trans fat–free) tortilla chips or SunChips
- 1 cup air-popped popcorn (no trans fat and not buttered)
- 1 graham cracker (2 squares or 1 rectangle)
- 1 cup low-fat chocolate milk (cold or hot)
- 3 Hershey's Kisses
- 15 jelly beans, gummy bears, or chocolate-covered raisins
- 20 M&M's or Reese's Pieces
- 2 Chocolate Meringue Cookies (page 244 or a commercial brand) or 1 small Coconut Macaroon (page 245 or a commercial brand)

Advance Prep Tips

Read through each week's menus ahead of time to plan your shopping and cooking according to your own schedule and habits. We've included "Convenience Notes," providing a heads-up for advance preparations. Whole grains cook themselves with very little help from you other than your remembering to turn off the stove when they're done. So we have you cooking them quite frequently in the evenings a day or two before they're needed for a recipe. You can also apply this strategy to cooked whole-grain cereal for breakfast, cooking it the night before and just heating it in a microwave in the morning—either at home or at work.

Don't Forget

▸ Try to drink a minimum of six 8-ounce glasses of water a day.
▸ Exercise or move for at least thirty minutes a day.
▸ Absolutely avoid high-calorie, sugar-sweetened beverages.
▸ Weigh yourself once a week—using the same scale, at the same time of day, and in the same clothes.
▸ Take a multivitamin every day.
▸ Eat slowly—taste and enjoy!

THE 21-DAY DIET
A THREE-WEEK CYCLE

See the Shopping Guide, starting on page 264, for all specifications for asterisked items.

DAY ONE

Breakfast

 1 cup sliced strawberries

 ⅔ cup yogurt*

 2 teaspoons sugar, jam, or honey, or non-caloric sweetener to taste (optional)

 1 slice whole-grain toast*

 1 tablespoon peanut butter (or other nut butter)

 Coffee or tea (with low-fat milk, if desired) (optional)

Lunch

 Delicate Spinach Soup (unlimited) (page 169)

 1 serving Ricotta Egg Salad (page 156)

 1 serving whole-grain crackers*

 Vegetables (unlimited) (any combination of baby carrots, bell pepper strips, celery sticks, cucumber slices, radishes, raw mushrooms, edible-pod peas, cauliflower, cherry tomatoes—and leftover cooked vegetables)

 1 medium apple

Snack

 1 serving Super Trail Mix (page 176)

Dinner

 Ten-Minute Tomato Soup (unlimited) (page 167)

 1 Baked Stuffed Pepper Filled with Bulgur–Pine Nut Pilaf (page 217)

 1 serving Protein-of-Choice (pages 201–210)

 2 tablespoons Tahini Sauce (page 191)

 Green salad (salad greens and vegetables) (unlimited)

 Buttermilk Ranch Dressing as needed (page 199)

 1 medium orange, cut into quarters

 2 Chocolate Meringue Cookies (page 244 or a commercial brand)

CONVENIENCE NOTE: Prepare Slow-Roasted Roma Tomatoes (page 223) to use on Days Two, Four, and whenever desired. Also, prepare Quick Marinated White Beans (page 163) and Pickled Red Onions (page 164)—and cook the mixed grains (page 243) for tomorrow night's dinner.

WEEK ONE

DAY TWO

Breakfast
1 tangerine, or half a medium orange

Scrambled Eggs with Broccoli and Cheddar (page 148)

Slow-Roasted Roma Tomatoes (unlimited, optional) (page 223)

1 teaspoon sugar or honey, or non-caloric sweetener to taste (optional)

Coffee or tea (with low-fat milk, if desired) (optional)

Lunch
Vegetable Broth with Corn (page 172) (unlimited)

Large spinach (unlimited) salad with:
   Raw mushrooms (unlimited)
   Shredded carrot (unlimited)
   Red onion (unlimited)
   Cherry tomatoes (unlimited)

3 tablespoons beans (any kind)

3 tablespoons crumbled feta, or ½ can tuna

¼ medium avocado, sliced or diced (about 4 healthy slices)

1 tablespoon sunflower seeds or nuts

Mollie's Vinaigrette as needed (page 198)

1 kiwi, sliced

Snack
1 serving Smoothie (pages 183–184, or up to 10 ounces of a commercial smoothie*)

Dinner
½ serving Protein-of-Choice (pages 201–210)

4 Broiled Baby Zucchini Boats with Parmesan Crust (page 236)

1 serving Quick Marinated White Beans (page 163)

Pickled Red Onions (unlimited) (page 164)

1 serving Mixed Grains with Cashews (page 243)

1 sliced peach with 3 tablespoons yogurt*

CONVENIENCE NOTE: Prepare Balsamic Glaze (page 193) for tomorrow night's dinner. You can also prepare the Broiled Eggplant, Bell Peppers, Onions, and Portobellos (page 235).

WEEK ONE

Breakfast

> 1 cup cooked whole-grain cereal*
>
> ½ medium apple, chopped (save the other half for lunch)
>
> ½ cup low-fat milk
>
> 1 teaspoon sugar or honey, or non-caloric sweetener to taste (optional)
>
> Coffee or tea (with low-fat milk, if desired) (optional)

Lunch

> Ethereal Broccoli Soup (unlimited) (page 168)
>
> 1 whole-wheat mini-pita (4-inch diameter or equivalent)
>
> 1 serving Quick Marinated White Beans (page 163) (left over from Day Two)
>
> Pickled Red Onions (page 164) (unlimited) (left over from Day Two)
>
> 2 tablespoons crumbled feta
>
> 4 olives
>
> Shredded romaine lettuce or spinach; chopped cucumber and tomato (unlimited)
>
> ½ cup red grapes and ½ medium apple, sliced (left over from breakfast)

Snack

> 1 serving Super Trail Mix (page 176)
>
> 1 tablespoon chocolate chips

Dinner

> 1 serving Protein-of-Choice (pages 201–210)
>
> Broiled Eggplant, Bell Peppers, Onions, and Portobellos (unlimited) (page 235)
>
> 2 tablespoons Balsamic Glaze (page 193)
>
> Green salad (salad greens and vegetables) (unlimited), tossed with ½ cup leftover Mixed Grains with Cashews (page 243)
>
> Honey-Mustard Dressing as needed (page 200)
>
> 1 medium peach or 2 small plums

WEEK ONE

DAY FOUR

Breakfast

    1 kiwi, sliced

    Scrambled Eggs with Spinach and Feta (page 148)

    Slow-Roasted Roma Tomatoes (unlimited) (page 223)

    1 teaspoon sugar or honey, or non-caloric sweetener to taste (optional)

    Coffee or tea (with low-fat milk, if desired) (optional)

Lunch

    ½ medium cantaloupe

    1 cup low-fat cottage cheese

    10 almonds or 1 tablespoon nut butter (any kind)

    1 tablespoon raisins

    1 slice whole-grain toast*

Snack

    Vegetables (unlimited) (any combination of baby carrots, bell pepper strips, celery sticks, cucumber slices, radishes, raw mushrooms, edible-pod peas, cauliflower, cherry tomatoes—and leftover cooked vegetables)

    3 tablespoons Honey-Mustard Dressing (page 200)

Dinner

    Vegetable Broth with White Beans (unlimited) (page 173)

    1½ cups cooked whole-grain pasta (dressed with 2 teaspoons olive oil)

    Tomato sauce (unlimited) (your own favorite homemade— or a commercial brand)

    ½ serving Protein-of-Choice (pages 201–210)—added to tomato sauce

    Italian-Style Pan-Sautéed Broccoli (unlimited) (page 232)

    Green salad (salad greens and vegetables) (unlimited)

    Creamy Balsamic Dressing as needed (page 199)

    1 cup sliced fresh pineapple (or ½ cup canned pineapple chunks, packed in juice)

Breakfast

    1 cup raspberries (fresh or unsweetened frozen, defrosted)

    1 cup cooked whole-grain cereal*

    ½ cup low-fat milk

    1 teaspoon sugar or honey, or non-caloric sweetener to taste (optional)

    Coffee or tea (with low-fat milk, if desired) (optional)

Lunch

    Vegetable Broth with Egg (unlimited) (page 172)

    Large romaine and mixed green (unlimited) salad with:

        ½ cup chickpeas or edamame (green soy beans)

        ¼ medium avocado, sliced or diced (about 4 healthy slices)

        2 tablespoons crumbled blue cheese or ½ can tuna

        Cherry tomatoes (unlimited)

        Red onion or scallion (unlimited)

        Cucumbers (unlimited)

    Creamy Balsamic Dressing as needed (page 199)

    1 medium orange

Snack

    1 serving Super Trail Mix (page 176)

    1 tablespoon chocolate chips

Dinner

    1 serving Protein-of-Choice (pages 201–210)

    Amazing Gravy as needed (page 196)

    1 serving Apple-Glazed Acorn Squash Rings (page 224)

    Braised Greens with Walnuts and Sour Cherries (unlimited) (page 231)

    ½ cup cooked whole-wheat orzo (rice-shaped pasta), drizzled with 1 teaspoon olive oil

    1 medium pear, sliced and drizzled with lemon

CONVENIENCE NOTE: Prepare Marinated Cucumbers (page 165) for tomorrow night's dinner.

WEEK ONE

DAY SIX

Breakfast

  1 serving Whole-Grain French Toast (page 153)

  1 tablespoon real maple syrup

  ½ cup blueberries (fresh or unsweetened frozen, defrosted)

  1 teaspoon sugar or honey, or non-caloric sweetener to taste (optional)

  Coffee or tea (with low-fat milk, if desired) (optional)

Lunch

  Vegetable Broth with Vermicelli and Peas (unlimited) (page 173)

  Burger—1 very lean beef or turkey burger (¼ pound raw weight),
    or 1 to 2 "veggie burgers"*

  1 whole-grain bun*

  2 tablespoons Avocado "Butter" (page 187) or Guacamole (page 186)

  Up to 1 tablespoon ketchup

  Up to 1 tablespoon mayonnaise

  Condiments (mustard, pickles, onions, lettuce, tomato, sauerkraut,
    tomato-based salsa) (unlimited)

  1 medium orange or 2 tangerines

Snack

  1 serving Smoothie (pages 183–184 or up to 10 ounces of a commercial
    smoothie*)

Dinner

  Miso Soup with Tofu and Scallions (unlimited) (page 170)

  1 serving Buckwheat Noodles with Cashews and Greens (page 216)

  ½ serving Protein-of-Choice (pages 201–210)

  Marinated Cucumbers (unlimited) (page 165)

  2 tangerines

  1 tablespoon chocolate chips

CONVENIENCE NOTE: You can prepare some of the ingredients for tomorrow night's Madras Vegetable Curry (page 214).

Breakfast

½ pink grapefruit

1 serving Miniature Frittata with Peas, Mint, and Goat Cheese (page 151)

1 teaspoon sugar or honey, or non-caloric sweetener to taste (optional)

Coffee or tea (with low-fat milk, if desired) (optional)

Lunch

Ten-Minute Tomato Soup (unlimited) (page 167)

1 serving Buckwheat Noodles with Cashews and Greens (page 216)
(left over from Day Six)

Marinated Cucumbers (unlimited) (page 165) (left over from Day Six)

10 strawberries

Snack

Vegetables (unlimited) (any combination of baby carrots, bell pepper strips, celery sticks, cucumber slices, radishes, raw mushrooms, edible-pod peas, cauliflower, cherry tomatoes—and leftover cooked vegetables)

3 tablespoons Avocado "Butter" (page 187) or Guacamole (page 186)

Tomato-based salsa (unlimited)

10 tortilla chips

Dinner

1 serving Madras Vegetable Curry (page 214)

½ serving Protein-of-Choice (pages 201–210)—added to curry

½ cup brown basmati rice

½ cup Spiced Yogurt (page 192)

1 tablespoon chopped, toasted almonds

1 tablespoon raisins

1 medium orange, sliced, and sprinkled with 1 tablespoon toasted unsweetened coconut

CONVENIENCE NOTE: Prepare Easy Three-Bean Chili (page 211) for tomorrow night's dinner.

WEEK ONE

DAY EIGHT

Breakfast

> 1 cup cooked whole-grain cereal*
>
> ½ medium apple, chopped (save the other half for lunch)
>
> 1 tablespoon chopped walnuts
>
> ½ cup low-fat milk
>
> 1 teaspoon sugar or honey, or non-caloric sweetener to taste (optional)
>
> Coffee or tea (with low-fat milk, if desired) (optional)

Lunch

> Vegetable Broth with Egg (unlimited) (page 172)
>
> Large spinach salad (unlimited) with tofu, chicken, tuna, or salmon
> (palm-size serving)
> 5 sliced, cooked beets (optional)
> Cucumber (unlimited)
> Shredded carrot (unlimited)
> Red onion (unlimited)
> Cherry tomatoes (unlimited)
>
> Roasted Garlic Vinaigrette as needed (page 198)
>
> ½ medium apple (left over from breakfast)

Snack

> ½ serving whole-grain crackers*
>
> 1 tablespoon peanut butter (or other nut butter)
>
> Vegetables (unlimited) (any combination of baby carrots, bell pepper strips,
> celery sticks, cucumber slices, radishes, raw mushrooms, edible-pod
> peas, cauliflower, cherry tomatoes—and leftover cooked vegetables)

Dinner

> 1 serving Easy Three-Bean Chili (page 211)
>
> ½ ounce cheddar cheese, grated (optional)
>
> 1 serving Bulgur with Olive Oil and Lemon (page 239)
>
> Green salad (salad greens and vegetables) (unlimited)
>
> Creamy Balsamic Dressing as needed (page 199)
>
> ½ medium peach with ½ cup yogurt*

CONVENIENCE NOTE: Prepare Roasted Vegetables (pages 226–228) for tomorrow night's dinner and for possible snacking. After the vegetables are done, turn down the oven and prepare Slow-Roasted Roma Tomatoes (page 223) for later this week. Also prepare Balsamic Glaze (page 193) and Millet and Quinoa with Toasted Sunflower Seeds (page 241) for tomorrow night's dinner.

DAY NINE

Breakfast

> ½ pink grapefruit
>
> Swiss Cheese, Mushroom, and Scallion Omelet (page 149)
>
> 1 teaspoon sugar or honey, or non-caloric sweetener to taste (optional)
>
> Coffee or tea (with low-fat milk, if desired) (optional)

Lunch

> 1 whole-wheat mini-pita (4-inch diameter or equivalent)
>
> Up to ⅓ cup Hummus (page 190 or a commercial brand)
>
> 4 olives
>
> Shredded lettuce (unlimited)
>
> Minced cucumbers (unlimited)
>
> Chopped tomatoes (unlimited)
>
> 2 tablespoons Tahini Sauce (page 191)
>
> 1 medium orange or 2 tangerines

Snack

> 1 serving Super Trail Mix (page 176)

Dinner

> Ten-Minute Tomato Soup (unlimited) (page 167)
>
> 1 serving Protein-of-Choice (pages 201–210)
>
> Roasted Vegetables—any single one, or a combination (unlimited) (pages 226–228)
>
> 1 serving Millet and Quinoa with Toasted Sunflower Seeds (page 241)
>
> Balsamic Glaze as needed (page 193)
>
> 1 medium apple, sliced and sprinkled with ½ teaspoon cinnamon-sugar

CONVENIENCE NOTE: Prepare Ricotta Egg Salad (page 156) or Tofu "Egg" Salad (page 157) for tomorrow's lunch; prepare Mediterranean-Style French Lentil Salad (page 161) for tomorrow's dinner and lunch the following day. You can also put together a batch of Baked Coated Nuts (pages 177 and 178).

WEEK TWO

DAY TEN

Breakfast

1 cup sliced fresh pineapple (or ½ cup canned pineapple chunks, packed in juice)

1 cup low-fat cottage cheese

1 slice whole-grain toast*

1 tablespoon peanut butter (or other nut butter)

1 teaspoon sugar or honey, or non-caloric sweetener to taste (optional)

Coffee or tea (with low-fat milk, if desired) (optional)

Lunch

Ten-Minute Tomato Soup (unlimited) (page 167)

1 serving Ricotta Egg Salad (page 156) or Tofu "Egg" Salad (page 157) on salad greens (unlimited)

1 serving whole-grain crackers*

Vegetables (unlimited) (any combination of baby carrots, bell pepper strips, celery sticks, cucumber slices, radishes, raw mushrooms, edible-pod peas, cauliflower, cherry tomatoes—and leftover cooked vegetables)

1 medium peach or 2 small plums

Snack

6 ounces yogurt*

1 serving Baked Coated Nuts (pages 177 and 178)

Dinner

Vegetable Broth with Vermicelli and Peas (unlimited) (page 173)

½ serving Protein-of-Choice (pages 201–210)

1 tablespoon Pomegranate-Lime Glaze (page 194)

1 serving Mediterranean-Style French Lentil Salad (page 161)

1 Sparkling Sweet Potato (page 225)

10 large strawberries dipped in 2 tablespoons melted chocolate chips

CONVENIENCE NOTE: Cook wheat berries for tomorrow night's soup.

WEEK TWO

DAY ELEVEN

Breakfast

1 cup raspberries (fresh or unsweetened frozen, defrosted)

Scrambled Eggs with Spinach (page 147)

1 teaspoon sugar or honey, or non-caloric sweetener to taste (optional)

Coffee or tea (with low-fat milk, if desired) (optional)

Lunch

Ethereal Broccoli Soup (unlimited) (page 168)

1 serving Mediterranean-Style French Lentil Salad (page 161)
(left over from Day Ten) on salad greens (unlimited)

1 serving whole-grain crackers*

1 medium orange

Snack

1 serving Super Trail Mix (page 176)

1 tablespoon chocolate chips

Dinner

Vegetable Broth with Wheat Berries (unlimited) (page 173)

1 serving Broiled Eggplant Parmesan (page 215)

Spinach with Pine Nuts and Raisins (unlimited) (page 230)

1 cup blackberries (fresh or unsweetened frozen, defrosted) with
½ cup yogurt*

CONVENIENCE NOTE: Cook barley for the Mushroom-Barley Burgers (page 212) you will have two nights from now—plus a little extra for the following day's soup. Prepare ingredients for Thai-Inspired Red or Green Curry (pages 221 or 222) and Marinated Cucumbers (page 165) for tomorrow night's dinner.

DAY TWELVE

Breakfast

    1 cup cooked whole-grain cereal*

    ½ cup low-fat milk

    3 dried apricots, sliced

    1 tablespoon chopped almonds

    1 teaspoon sugar or honey, or non-caloric sweetener to taste (optional)

    Coffee or tea (with low-fat milk, if desired) (optional)

Lunch

    Vegetable Broth with Wheat Berries (unlimited) (page 173)

    Nachos Lunch (page 158)

    Green salad (salad greens plus vegetables) (unlimited)

    Mollie's Vinaigrette as needed (page 198)

Snack

    1 medium apple

    1 serving Baked Coated Nuts (pages 177 and 178)

Dinner

    1 serving Thai-inspired Green or Red Curry (pages 221 or 222)

    1 serving Protein-of-Choice (pages 201–210)—added to curry

    ½ cup brown basmati rice

    Marinated Cucumbers (unlimited) (page 165)

    ½ mango, sliced (about 6 slices) and sprinkled with fresh lime juice

CONVENIENCE NOTE: Prepare the mixture for Mushroom-Barley Burgers (page 212) for tomorrow night's dinner.

Breakfast

    1 serving Whole-Grain French Toast (page 153)

    1 tablespoon real maple syrup

    1 cup sliced strawberries

    1 teaspoon sugar or honey, or non-caloric sweetener to taste (optional)

    Coffee or tea (with low-fat milk, if desired)

Lunch

    Ten-Minute Tomato Soup (unlimited) (page 167)

    Large spinach (unlimited) salad with:
        Raw mushrooms (unlimited)
        Shredded carrot (unlimited)
        Red onion (unlimited)
        Cherry tomatoes (unlimited)
        ¼ medium avocado, sliced or diced (about 4 healthy slices)
        3 tablespoons beans (any kind)
        3 tablespoons crumbled feta or ½ can tuna

    Honey-Mustard Dressing as needed (page 200)

    1 serving whole-grain crackers*

Snack

    1 serving Super Trail Mix (page 176)

    1 or 2 kiwis, sliced

Dinner

    1 Mushroom-Barley Burger (page 212)

    Tomato-based salsa (unlimited)

    Five-Minute Flash-Cooked Green Beans (unlimited) (page 234)

    Spaghetti Squash (unlimited) (page 233)

    ½ cup fruit sorbet

DAY FOURTEEN

Breakfast

A 3-inch wedge of honeydew sprinkled with fresh lime juice

1 serving Miniature Frittata with Artichoke Hearts and Parmesan (page 150)

1 teaspoon sugar or honey, or non-caloric sweetener to taste (optional)

Coffee or tea (with low-fat milk, if desired) (optional)

Lunch

Vegetable Broth with Mushrooms and Barley (unlimited) (page 172)

Burger—1 very lean beef or turkey burger (¼ pound raw weight), or 1 to 2 "veggie burgers"*

1 whole-grain bun*

2 tablespoons Avocado "Butter" (page 187) or Guacamole (page 186)

Up to 1 tablespoon ketchup

Up to 1 tablespoon mayonnaise

Condiments (mustard, pickles, lettuce, tomato, sauerkraut, tomato-based salsa) (unlimited)

1 medium orange

Snack

Chocolate-Banana Shake (page 184)

Dinner

Delicate Spinach Soup (unlimited) (page 169)

1 serving Vegetable-Almond Fried Rice (page 220)

1 serving Honey-Broiled Pears (page 246) with ½ cup yogurt*

CONVENIENCE NOTE: Prepare Gazpacho (page 174) for tomorrow's lunch.

Breakfast

> ½ pink grapefruit
>
> Scrambled Eggs with Broccoli (page 148)
>
> 1 teaspoon sugar or honey, or non-caloric sweetener to taste (optional)
>
> Coffee or tea (with low-fat milk, if desired) (optional)

Lunch

> Gazpacho (unlimited) (page 174)
>
> Broiled Open-Face Cheddar Sandwich (page 156)
>
> Vegetables (unlimited) (any combination of baby carrots, bell pepper strips, celery sticks, cucumber slices, radishes, raw mushrooms, edible-pod peas, cauliflower, cherry tomatoes—and leftover cooked vegetables)
>
> 3 tablespoons Buttermilk Ranch Dressing (page 199)
>
> 1 medium apple

Snack

> 1 serving Super Trail Mix (page 176)
>
> 1 tablespoon chocolate chips

Dinner

> Vegetable Broth with White Beans (unlimited) (page 173)
>
> 1 serving Protein-of-Choice (pages 201–210)
>
> Sesame-Mustard Glaze as needed (page 194)
>
> 1 serving Whole-Wheat Couscous with Pistachios and Orange Zest (page 238)
>
> Zucchini and Sweet Onions in Butter-Spiked Olive Oil (unlimited) (page 237)
>
> 2 small plums, sliced and drizzled with fresh lemon juice

WEEK THREE

DAY SIXTEEN

Breakfast

Fruit platter:
   1 kiwi, sliced
   ½ cup blueberries (fresh or unsweetened frozen, defrosted)
   ½ medium banana, sliced
1 cup low-fat cottage cheese or ⅔ cup yogurt*
1 slice whole-grain toast*
1 tablespoon peanut butter (or other nut butter)
1 teaspoon sugar or honey, or non-caloric sweetener to taste (optional)
Coffee or tea (with low-fat milk, if desired) (optional)

Lunch

2 Portobello Pizzas (page 159)
1 whole-grain English muffin* (both halves, toasted)
Green salad (salad greens and vegetables) (unlimited)
Creamy Balsamic Dressing as needed (page 199)
1 medium orange or 2 tangerines

Snack

Up to ⅓ cup Tangy Black-Bean Dip (page 189) or ¼ cup Hummus (page 190 or a commercial brand)
Vegetables (unlimited) (any combination of baby carrots, bell pepper strips, celery sticks, cucumber slices, radishes, raw mushrooms, edible-pod peas, cauliflower, cherry tomatoes—and leftover cooked vegetables)
10 tortilla chips

Dinner

1½ cups cooked whole-grain pasta (dressed with 2 teaspoons olive oil)
Tomato sauce (unlimited) (your own favorite homemade—or a commercial brand)
½ serving Protein-of-Choice (pages 201–210)—added to tomato sauce
Italian-Style Pan-Sautéed Broccoli (unlimited) (page 232)
Green Salad (salad greens and vegetables) (unlimited)
Creamy Balsamic Dressing as needed (page 199)
Cantaloupe slices sprinkled with fresh lemon juice (unlimited)

CONVENIENCE NOTE: Prepare Slow-Roasted Roma Tomatoes (page 223) for tomorrow and for later this week. Also prepare Amazing Mushroom Gravy (page 197) and Kasha Varnishkes (page 242) for tomorrow night's dinner.

DAY SEVENTEEN

Breakfast

    1 cup cooked whole-grain cereal*

    ½ cup low-fat milk

    2 dried plums or figs

    1 teaspoon sugar or honey, or non-caloric sweetener to taste (optional)

    Coffee or tea (with low-fat milk, if desired) (optional)

Lunch

    Ten-Minute Tomato Soup (unlimited) (page 167)

    Large spinach (unlimited) salad with
        Raw mushrooms (unlimited)
        Shredded carrot (unlimited)
        Red onion (unlimited)
        Cherry tomatoes (unlimited)
        ¼ medium avocado, sliced or diced (about 4 healthy slices)
        1 hard-boiled egg
        3 tablespoons beans (any kind)
        3 tablespoons crumbled feta or ½ can tuna

    Mollie's Vinaigrette as needed (page 198)

Snack

    Chocolate-Banana Shake (page 184)

Dinner

    1 serving Protein-of-Choice (pages 201–210)

    Amazing Mushroom Gravy as needed (page 197)

    1 serving Kasha Varnishkes (page 242)

    Roasted Brussels Sprouts (unlimited) (page 228)

    Slow-Roasted Roma Tomatoes (unlimited) (page 223)

    1 medium orange, sliced, with 1 tablespoon toasted unsweetened coconut

CONVENIENCE NOTE: Prepare Black Beans with Exotic Fruit (page 162) for tomorrow night's dinner.

DAY EIGHTEEN

Breakfast

2 fried eggs (fried in 1 teaspoon butter or oil)

1 slice Canadian bacon (meat or soy-based)

One-Minute Spinach (unlimited) (page 229)

Slow-Roasted Roma Tomatoes (unlimited) (page 223)

½ whole-grain English muffin* with 1 teaspoon butter or olive oil

1 teaspoon sugar or honey, or non-caloric sweetener to taste (optional)

Coffee or tea (with low-fat milk, if desired) (optional)

Lunch

½ medium cantaloupe

1 cup low-fat cottage cheese

1 tablespoon dried cranberries

½ whole-grain English muffin (the half left over from breakfast)

1 tablespoon peanut butter (or other nut butter)

Snack

1 serving Super Trail Mix (page 176)

1 tablespoon chocolate chips

Dinner

1 serving Black Beans with Exotic Fruit (page 162)

½ serving Protein-of-Choice (pages 201–210)

1 serving Roasted Butternut Squash (page 226)

2 tablespoons Pomegranate-Lime Glaze (page 194)

Green salad (salad greens and vegetables) (unlimited)

Roasted Garlic Vinaigrette as needed (page 198)

1 cup watermelon chunks, sprinkled with fresh lime juice

CONVENIENCE NOTE: Cook wild rice for tomorrow night's dinner and the next day's soup (page 55).

WEEK THREE

Breakfast

> 1 cup cooked whole-grain cereal*
>
> ½ cup low-fat milk
>
> 1 medium peach
>
> 1 teaspoon sugar or honey, or non-caloric sweetener to taste (optional)
>
> Coffee or tea (with low-fat milk, if desired) (optional)

Lunch

> 1 serving Black Beans with Exotic Fruit (page 162) (left over from Day Eighteen)
>
> 1 steamed corn tortilla
>
> 2 tablespoons Avocado "Butter" (page 187) or Guacamole (page 186)

Snack

> 1 serving whole-grain crackers
>
> 1 tablespoon peanut butter (or other nut butter)
>
> Vegetables (unlimited) (any combination of baby carrots, bell pepper strips, celery sticks, cucumber slices, radishes, raw mushrooms, edible-pod peas, cauliflower, cherry tomatoes—and leftover cooked vegetables)

Dinner

> Ten-Minute Tomato Soup (unlimited) (page 167)
>
> 1 serving Protein-of-Choice (pages 201–210)
>
> Roasted Asparagus (unlimited) (page 227)
>
> ½ cup wild rice (page 55) with 1 tablespoon each chopped hazelnuts and dried cranberries
>
> Green salad (salad greens with vegetables) (unlimited)
>
> Mollie's Vinaigrette as needed (page 198)
>
> 1 kiwi, sliced
>
> 2 Chocolate Meringue Cookies (page 244 or a commercial brand)

CONVENIENCE NOTE: Prepare Taboo-less Tabouleh (page 166) for tomorrow's lunch.

WEEK THREE

DAY TWENTY

Breakfast

> 1 serving Whole-Grain French Toast (page 153)
>
> 1 tablespoon real maple syrup
>
> ½ cup blackberries (fresh or unsweetened frozen, defrosted)
>
> 1 teaspoon sugar or honey, or non-caloric sweetener to taste (optional)
>
> Coffee or tea (with low-fat milk, if desired) (optional)

Lunch

> Vegetable Broth with Wild Rice (unlimited) (page 173)
>
> 1 serving Taboo-less Tabouleh (page 166)
>
> 2 tablespoons Tahini Sauce (page 191)
>
> 1 medium pear
>
> ½ serving Baked Coated Nuts (pages 177 and 178)

Snack

> 1 serving Smoothie (pages 183–184 or up to 10 ounces of a commercial smoothie*)

Dinner

> 1 serving Protein-of-Choice (pages 201–210), cut into strips
>
> ½ cup pinto beans
>
> 2 tablespoons Avocado "Butter" (page 187) or Guacamole (page 186)
>
> Tomato-based salsa (unlimited)
>
> 1 steamed corn tortilla
>
> Green salad (salad greens with vegetables) (unlimited)
>
> Buttermilk Ranch Dressing as needed (page 199)
>
> 10 strawberries dipped in 2 tablespoons melted chocolate chips

WEEK THREE

Breakfast

    1 serving Miniature Frittata with Zucchini, Herbs, and Feta (page 152)

    1 medium peach or 2 small plums

    1 teaspoon sugar or honey, or non-caloric sweetener to taste (optional)

    Coffee or tea (with low-fat milk, if desired) (optional)

Lunch

    Delicate Spinach Soup (unlimited) (page 169)

    1 serving Avocado Waldorf (page 160)

    1 serving whole-grain crackers*

Snack

    Up to ⅓ cup Tangy Black-Bean Dip (page 189) or ¼ cup Hummus (page 190 or a commercial brand)

    Vegetables (unlimited) (any combination of baby carrots, bell pepper strips, celery sticks, cucumber slices, radishes, raw mushrooms, edible-pod peas, cauliflower, cherry tomatoes—and leftover cooked vegetables)

Dinner

    Vegetable Broth with Egg (unlimited) (page 172)

    1 serving Green Beans in Crunchy Peanut Coating with Protein-of-Choice (page 218)

    ½ cup brown rice

    ½ cup raspberries (fresh or unsweetened frozen, defrosted) with ½ cup yogurt*

WEEK THREE

13

The
Portable Plan

MAYBE YOU ARE a busy college student who sees a kitchen only three times a year. Perhaps you are a teenager, hanging out with friends when not in school—loaded down with homework, or running to an after-school job or sports practice. Or you're traveling for work, and grabbing your meals out of supermarkets to save time and money. Whatever your circumstances, know that you are not alone. Many of us need a portable "Plan B," at least some of the time. So here is a very simple plan based mostly on ready-to-eat fare procurable from just about any grocery store with a decent deli and a reasonably good salad bar.

The Portable Plan lays out four very simple meals a day: breakfast, two "lunch-snacks," and dinner. Try to eat these meals approximately three hours apart, limiting each one to a single sitting, rather than grazing. Drink lots of water in between. You may have one alcoholic drink (not sugar-sweetened) daily, if you wish.

Follow the Portable Plan for a week and then repeat it if you wish. After two weeks, you can take a few days off to eat just normally (whatever that means to you) and then, if you like, go back on for another week or two or three—until you reach your desired weight goal. Clearly, this plan is very limited, but it is easy to follow and nutritionally balanced. (Don't forget to drink lots of water and take your daily multivitamin!)

Read through Chapter 15 (page 249) before you begin. There you will find more detailed ideas for navigating ethnic restaurants, salad bars, delis, diners, and fast-food joints, as well as a section called How to Eat on the Go While Managing Your Weight.

The dinners in these menus are interchangeable. You can trade one for another at your convenience, depending on what's available. Also, although coffee and tea are suggested at breakfast only, feel free to drink them throughout the day if you wish, as long as you don't shortchange your intake of water.

DAY ONE

Breakfast

Up to 4 cups cut-up fresh fruit (melon, apples, berries, plums, peaches, pineapple, kiwi, 1 medium banana)

2 tablespoons nuts

1 cup low-fat milk

Coffee or tea (optional)

1 teaspoon sugar or honey, or non-caloric sweetener to taste (optional)

Lunch-Snack 1

Up to 2 good-quality protein bars*

Lunch-Snack 2

⅓ cup Hummus (page 190 or a commercial brand)

Vegetables (unlimited) (any combination of baby carrots, bell pepper strips, celery sticks, cucumber slices, radishes, raw mushrooms, edible-pod peas, cauliflower, cherry tomatoes—and cooked vegetables)

1 serving whole-grain crackers*

Dinner

Vegetable Broth (unlimited) (see pages 171–173) or 1 cup non-creamy soup

1 serving whole-grain bread*

1 serving Protein-of-Choice (see pages 201–210)

Tomato-based salsa as needed

Green salad (salad greens with vegetables) (unlimited)

Salad dressing of choice—or olive oil and vinegar—as needed

THE PORTABLE PLAN

DAY TWO

Breakfast
- 1 cup cooked oatmeal or whole-grain cereal (hot or cold)*
- 1 tablespoon raisins
- 1 teaspoon sugar or honey, or non-caloric sweetener to taste (optional)
- 1 cup low-fat milk
- Coffee or tea (optional)

Lunch-Snack 1
- Up to three 4-ounce yogurts or two 6-ounce yogurts*

Lunch-Snack 2
- 1 serving Super Trail Mix (see pages 175–176)
- Fresh fruit as desired

Dinner
- Burger—1 very lean beef or turkey burger (¼ pound raw weight), or 1 to 2 "veggie burgers"*
- 1 whole-grain bun*
- Up to 1 tablespoon ketchup
- Up to 1 tablespoon mayonnaise
- Condiments (mustard, pickles, onions, lettuce, tomato, sauerkraut, tomato-based salsa) (unlimited)
- Green salad (salad greens with vegetables) (unlimited)
- Salad dressing of choice—or olive oil and vinegar—as needed

n

DAY THREE

Breakfast

1 slice whole-grain toast with 1 teaspoon butter or olive oil

1 serving MicroEggs (page 154) or 2 hard-boiled eggs with One-Minute Spinach (page 229)

Coffee or tea (with low-fat milk, if desired) (optional)

1 teaspoon sugar or honey, or non-caloric sweetener to taste (optional)

Lunch-Snack 1

Up to 4 cups cut-up fresh fruit (melon, apples, berries, plums, peaches, pineapple, 1 medium banana)

1 cup low-fat milk

Coffee or tea (optional)

1 teaspoon sugar or honey, or non-caloric sweetener to taste (optional)

Lunch-Snack 2

2 tablespoons peanut butter (or other nut butter)

1 serving whole-grain crackers*

Vegetables (unlimited) (any combination of baby carrots, bell pepper strips, celery sticks, cucumber slices, radishes, raw mushrooms, edible-pod peas, cauliflower, cherry tomatoes—and cooked vegetables)

Dinner

Vegetable broth (unlimited) (page 171) or 1 cup non-creamy soup

1½ cups stewed tomatoes (canned) with 1 tablespoon olive oil

1 serving Protein-of-Choice (pages 201–210)

Green salad (salad greens and vegetables) (unlimited)

Salad dressing of choice—or olive oil and vinegar—as needed

THE PORTABLE PLAN

DAY FOUR

Breakfast

    1 cup cooked oatmeal or whole-grain cereal (hot or cold)*

    1 tablespoon dried cranberries

    1 tablespoon chopped walnuts

    1 cup low-fat milk

    Coffee or tea (optional)

    1 teaspoon sugar or honey, or non-caloric sweetener to taste (optional)

Lunch-Snack 1

    Up to 2 good-quality protein bars*

Lunch-Snack 2

    ½ medium cantaloupe

    1 cup low-fat cottage cheese

    1 tablespoon raisins

    10 almonds

Dinner

    1½ cups vegetarian chili (from a can—or use the recipe on page 211)

    1 ounce Cheddar or mozzarella cheese (1 stick)

    Green salad (salad greens and vegetables) (unlimited)

    Salad dressing of choice—or olive oil and vinegar—as needed

    1 serving whole-grain crackers*

DAY FIVE

Breakfast

Up to 4 cups cut-up fresh fruit (melon, apples, berries, plums, peaches, pineapple, kiwi, 1 medium banana)

2 pieces whole-grain toast*

2 tablespoons peanut butter (or other nut butter)

Coffee or tea (with low-fat milk, if desired) (optional)

1 teaspoon sugar or honey, or non-caloric sweetener to taste (optional)

Lunch-Snack 1

Up to three 4-ounce yogurts or two 6-ounce yogurts*

Lunch-Snack 2

1 serving Super Trail Mix (pages 175–176)

Fresh fruit as desired

Dinner

Up to 1 cup cooked lean ground beef or turkey—or 2 "veggie burgers," crumbled*

2 cups cooked pasta (whole wheat, if available)

Tomato sauce (your favorite kind) (unlimited)

Cooked vegetables (not potatoes) with olive oil, salt, and pepper (unlimited)

Green salad (salad greens and vegetables) (unlimited)

Salad dressing of choice—or olive oil and vinegar—as needed

THE PORTABLE PLAN

Breakfast

    1 cup cooked oatmeal or whole-grain cereal (hot or cold)*

    1 tablespoon raisins

    1 cup low-fat milk

    Coffee or tea (optional)

    1 teaspoon sugar or honey, or non-caloric sweetener to taste (optional)

Lunch-Snack 1

    Up to ⅓ cup Hummus (page 190 or a commercial brand)

    1 serving whole-grain crackers*

    Vegetables (unlimited) (any combination of baby carrots, bell pepper strips, celery sticks, cucumber slices, radishes, raw mushrooms, edible-pod peas, cauliflower, cherry tomatoes—and cooked vegetables)

Lunch-Snack 2

    2 medium apples

    ¼ cup nuts

Dinner

    Vegetable broth (unlimited) (pages 171–173) or 1 cup non-creamy soup

    1½ cups stewed tomatoes (canned) with 1 tablespoon olive oil

    1 serving Protein-of-Choice (pages 201–210)

    Green salad (salad greens and vegetables) (unlimited)

    Salad dressing of choice—or olive oil and vinegar—as needed

THE PORTABLE PLAN

Breakfast

1 slice whole-grain toast with 1 teaspoon butter or olive oil

1 serving MicroEggs (page 154) or 2 hard-boiled eggs with One-Minute Spinach (page 229)

Coffee or tea (with low-fat milk, if desired) (optional)

1 teaspoon sugar or honey, or non-caloric sweetener to taste (optional)

Lunch-Snack 1

1 serving Super Trail Mix (pages 175–176)

Lunch-Snack 2

2 medium apples

1 ounce Cheddar or mozzarella cheese (1 stick)

Dinner

Burger—1 very lean beef or turkey burger (¼ pound raw weight)—or 1 to 2 "veggie burgers"*

1 whole-grain bun*

Up to 1 tablespoon ketchup

Up to 1 tablespoon mayonnaise

Condiments (mustard, pickles, onions, lettuce, tomato, sauerkraut, tomato-based salsa) (unlimited)

Green salad (salad greens with vegetables) (unlimited)

Salad dressing of choice—or olive oil and vinegar—as needed

THE PORTABLE PLAN

14

Lifelong Maintenance

Y OU HAVE LOST the weight you hoped to lose and have arrived at
your healthy goal. Bravo! Now what?

Your relationship with food is on a new track, and your streamlined
body is something you are happy with and want to preserve. The chal-
lenge is to stay here, on this shore, where all the dots have been connected and you have the tools you need—the facts, science, recipes, and
encouragement.

You will now be your own monitor of healthy weight status and this
might involve some trial and error. You have what you need to keep
going and to find and customize the comfort zone that is uniquely yours.

Here are some guidelines:

▶ Stay with the Nine Turning Points:

1. Eat lots of vegetables and fruits.
2. Say yes to good fats.
3. Upgrade your carbohydrates.
4. Choose healthy proteins.
5. Stay hydrated.
6. Drink alcohol in moderation (optional).
7. Take a multivitamin every day.
8. Move more.
9. Eat mindfully all day long.

- Keep going with three meals plus one or two snacks daily, if needed.
- Continue spreading out your eating over the course of each day, rather than reverting to erratic patterns of starvation and gorging.
- You can begin to add in some extra things. (For example, add a piece of whole-grain toast to the egg breakfasts, if you wish.) The best foods to increase are
  - Pure proteins (chicken, fish, tofu, nonfat yogurt)
  - Fruit
  - Vegetables
  - Nuts
- Keep tabs on portion size. This is not just for when you're "on a diet"; it's something to always be aware of. Over time, portion-size awareness will become second nature to you.
- Stop eating when you are *comfortable* and *well before you are stuffed*.
- Expand your cooking repertoire and experiment with some new dishes.
- Have dessert, but limit it to every *other* night. *Or* add one snack a couple of times a week—something that you have missed and that brings you satisfaction.
- You may have up to two alcoholic drinks a day, if you wish. Try to avoid sugary or highly caloric mixed drinks.
- Let dinner end your eating for the day. Get into the habit of brushing your teeth after dinner, as this will help. If you're a little hungry at bedtime, let the slight discomfort be an overnight bridge connecting you with a delicious breakfast. Over time, this hunger pattern should dissipate if you are eating well.
- Keep up the full daily intake of water.
- Ideally, you have been doing your resistance and calorie-burning exercises and you'll continue doing them forever. These will keep your metabolism primed.
- Pay close attention to the information in Chapter 15 (page 249). This will help you navigate the big, wide world.
- Continue weighing yourself once a week at the same time of day and in the same clothing. This is very important, as it will be your indicator of weight maintenance—the truest way to know if your choices are serving you well. If your weight starts to creep back up, you'll need to trouble-shoot your intake. Cut back a little (less wine? fewer desserts?) and/or ramp up your physical activity (add an extra fifteen-minute walk every day for a week, if you can). Nipping here, tucking there—this is all a work in progress! And you can always go back on the 21-Day Diet for another three weeks if you need to.

Your Food Budget—Live Within Your Means

The best maintenance advice we can give you is this: Get into the habit of calculating trade-offs. Come to view "treats" as a limited commodity— limited for very technical reasons—rather than as something morally and psychologically loaded. It's like making a budget. Spend within your means.

So, without going into obsessive mode, just figure out before, say, a dinner in a restaurant, that you can afford either wine or a mixed cocktail, but not both. And if you get a drink (or two), perhaps that gets traded against having a whole dessert (you can still have two bites of someone else's). Decide on bread *or* rice *or* potato. You get the idea.

Many people find it helpful simply to have one day a week when they can eat all they want. Others get the satisfaction they need from knowing they can have one or two glasses of wine daily and a single helping of dessert every other day (as in the Warm-Up Plan). Above all, remember to enjoy your food, whatever you're eating! How you find, define, and come to peace with your own food happiness is something you will figure out—and modify—all through your life. We hope that journey will be a long and happy one.

The Recipes

Scrambled Eggs with Spinach

There's an easy way to "green-light" even the dreariest weekday morning!

2 large eggs
Salt
Freshly ground black pepper
Nonstick spray
½ teaspoon extra-virgin
   olive oil
1 large handful spinach (about
   2 ounces), minced
½ teaspoon butter

▶ YIELD: 1 SERVING

Protein: 143 g / Saturated Fat: 5 g /
Polyunsaturated Fat: 2 g /
Monounsaturated Fat: 6 g /
Dietary Fiber: 1 g / Calories: 198

1. Place an 8- or 10-inch nonstick omelet pan or regular frying pan over medium heat.

2. In small bowl, beat the eggs until smooth, adding a pinch of salt and a grind or two of black pepper.

3. When the pan has been heating for about a minute, spray it lightly with nonstick spray and add the olive oil, swirling to coat the pan. Turn up the heat to high and add the spinach and another pinch of salt. Cook for about 1 minute over high heat, until the spinach is wilted. Transfer to a plate (it can be the one you'll be eating from) and return the pan to the stove.

4. Turn the heat back down to medium and wait about 30 seconds, then add the butter. It should sizzle, then settle down. Tilt the pan in all directions to distribute the butter.

5. Quickly pour in the beaten eggs. As they begin to set, push the curds from the bottom to one side, allowing uncooked egg to flow into contact with the pan. After about 10 seconds, add the cooked spinach, as you continue pushing curds to the side as they form and puff.

6. As soon as the eggs stop flowing, you can flip them over for a few seconds to cook on the other side—or, if you like your eggs soft, just push them onto the plate and serve right away.

Scrambled Eggs with Spinach and Feta

Protein: 16 g / Saturated Fat: 7 g /
Polyunsaturated Fat: 2 g /
Monounsaturated Fat: 7 g /
Dietary Fiber: 1 g /Calories: 235

Follow the recipe for Scrambled Eggs with Spinach (previous page), including 1½ tablespoons crumbled feta cheese when you add the cooked spinach to the eggs in step 5.

Scrambled Eggs with Broccoli

Protein: 14 g / Saturated Fat: 5 g /
Polyunsaturated Fat: 2 g /
Monounsaturated Fat: 6 g /
Dietary Fiber: 1 g / Calories: 194

Follow the recipe for Scrambled Eggs with Spinach (previous page), replacing the spinach with a heaping ½ cup (or more, if you like) minced broccoli florets. The broccoli will take up to a minute longer to cook than the spinach.

Scrambled Eggs with Broccoli and Cheddar

Protein: 16 g / Saturated Fat: 5 g /
Polyunsaturated Fat: 2 g /
Monounsaturated Fat: 6 g /
Dietary Fiber: 1 g / Calories: 213

Prepare Scrambled Eggs with Broccoli as directed, including 1½ tablespoons grated low-fat sharp Cheddar when you add the cooked broccoli in step 5.

Swiss Cheese, Mushroom, and Scallion Omelet

In this simple omelet, the small touches of cheese, mushroom, and scallion go a long way. The tiny amounts of olive oil and butter add up flavor-wise, too.

2 large eggs
Salt
Freshly ground black pepper
Nonstick spray
½ teaspoon extra-virgin olive oil
½ teaspoon butter
4 or 5 medium-size mushrooms, thinly sliced
1 scallion, thinly sliced (include the green part)
1½ tablespoons grated Gruyère or Emmenthaler cheese

- *In a perfect world you will have remembered to warm the serving plate ahead of time in a microwave. Although not essential, this is a very nice touch.*

- *Have all the ingredients prepared and within reach before you begin cooking the omelet. Once you begin, this goes quickly.*

▶ **YIELD: 1 SERVING**
Protein: 18 g / Saturated Fat: 7 g /
Polyunsaturated Fat: 2 g /
Monounsaturated Fat: 7 g /
Dietary Fiber: 2 g / Calories: 254

1. Place an 8-inch nonstick omelet pan over medium heat.
2. In a small bowl, beat the eggs until smooth, adding a pinch of salt and a grind or two of black pepper.
3. When the pan has been heating for about a minute, spray it lightly with nonstick spray and add the olive oil, swirling to coat the pan. Turn up the heat to medium-high, and add the mushrooms and scallion, along with another pinch of salt. Cook for about 2 minutes over high heat, until the mushrooms turn a light golden brown. Scrape this mixture onto a plate (it can be the one you'll be eating from) and return the pan to the stove.
4. Turn the heat back down to medium, and wait about 30 seconds, then add the butter. It should sizzle, then settle down. Tilt the pan in all directions to distribute the butter, then pour in the egg mixture, keeping the heat at medium.
5. As the eggs begin to set at the edges, carefully push the cooked portion toward the center of the pan with a small spatula. At the same time, tilt the pan, allowing any remaining raw egg to fill the spaces.
6. As soon as the eggs stop flowing, you can flip the omelet to the other side if you like it drier, or just leave it on the first side if you like it soft. In either case, add the cooked mushroom mixture, distributing it over the surface, then sprinkle on the cheese.
7. Use the spatula to fold the omelet in half, and slide or flip it onto the waiting plate.

Miniature Frittata with Artichoke Hearts and Parmesan

A frittata is an oven-finished Italian-style omelet, filled with vegetables and cheese. It doesn't take much more work than a regular, French-style omelet, but can feel like more of a special-occasion item. Use a 6-inch nonstick frying pan with an ovenproof handle. Don't forget the oven mitt or pot holder.

4 large eggs

3 tablespoons grated Parmesan cheese

Salt

Freshly ground black pepper

2 teaspoons extra-virgin olive oil

6 artichoke hearts, thinly sliced

3 tablespoons finely minced red onion

½ teaspoon minced or crushed garlic

- *If you are using frozen artichoke hearts, defrost them first. If using canned hearts, drain them well.*

- *A good quality Parmesan cheese makes a big difference. Freshly (or recently) grated is ideal!*

- *This makes 2 servings. If you are cooking for one, keep in mind that it tastes very good leftover at room temperature.*

▶ **YIELD: 2 SERVINGS**
Protein: 18 g / Saturated Fat: 5 g / Polyunsaturated Fat: 2 g / Monounsaturated Fat: 8 g / Dietary Fiber: 5 g / Calories: 267

1. Preheat the broiler to 500°F and move the oven rack to the highest position.

2. In a medium bowl, whisk the eggs until smooth, then stir in 1½ tablespoons of the Parmesan, along with a pinch or two of salt and a few grinds of pepper. Set aside.

3. Place the pan over medium heat and wait 1 minute. Add the oil and swirl to coat the pan. Add the artichoke hearts, onion, and another pinch of salt. Sauté for 2 to 3 minutes, then add the garlic.

4. Pour in the egg mixture and let it sit still over the heat for about 30 seconds, then gently lift the edges with a spatula, and tilt the pan in all directions to let the loose egg move toward the edges. Allow it to sit for 5 minutes, until just about set. The top will still be wet.

5. Sprinkle on the remaining cheese, then transfer the pan to the broiler and broil for 2 to 3 minutes, or until the top is golden.

6. Using an oven mitt or pot holder, carefully remove the pan from the broiler, and let the frittata sit for about a minute to set. Loosen the edges with a spatula and transfer (sliding or flipping it) to a plate. Serve hot, warm, or at room temperature.

Miniature Frittata with Peas, Mint, and Goat Cheese

Fresh mint leaves are a wonderful, bright surprise and they go particularly well with the goat cheese. The peas make this beautiful. Use a 6-inch nonstick frying pan with an ovenproof handle. Don't forget the oven mitt or pot holder.

4 large eggs

3 tablespoons crumbled fresh goat cheese

2 tablespoons minced fresh mint leaves

Salt

Freshly ground black pepper

2 teaspoons extra-virgin olive oil

3 tablespoons finely minced scallion

¾ cup peas (frozen/defrosted)

½ teaspoon minced garlic

- *A quick way to defrost frozen peas is to place them in a strainer and rinse them under lukewarm running water for a minute or less. Shake dry, then pat with paper towels.*

- *This makes 2 servings. If you are cooking for one, keep in mind that it tastes very good leftover at room temperature.*

▶ **YIELD: 2 SERVINGS**
Protein: 18 g / Saturated Fat: 6 g /
Polyunsaturated Fat: 2 g /
Monounsaturated Fat: 8 g /
Dietary Fiber: 2 g / Calories: 277

1. Preheat the broiler to 500°F and move the oven rack to the highest position.

2. In a medium bowl, whisk the eggs until smooth, then stir in 1½ tablespoons of the goat cheese, along with the mint, a pinch or two of salt, and a few grinds of pepper. Set aside.

3. Place the pan over medium heat and wait 1 minute. Add the oil and swirl to coat the pan. Add the scallion and peas, along with another pinch of salt. Sauté for about 2 minutes, then stir in the garlic.

4. Pour in the egg mixture and let it sit still over the heat for about 30 seconds, then gently lift the edges with a spatula, and tilt the pan in all directions to let the loose egg move toward the edges. Allow it to sit for 5 minutes, until just about set. The top will still be wet.

5. Sprinkle on the remaining cheese, then transfer the pan to the broiler and broil for 2 to 3 minutes, or until the top is golden.

6. Using an oven mitt or pot holder, carefully remove the pan from the broiler, and let the frittata sit for about a minute to set. Loosen the edges with a spatula and transfer (sliding or flipping it) to a plate. Serve hot, warm, or at room temperature.

Miniature Frittata with Zucchini, Herbs, and Feta

The overlapping circles of zucchini look lovely in this light but satisfying breakfast dish. Fresh cherry tomatoes in season (or Slow-Roasted Roma Tomatoes, page 223) are the perfect accompaniment. Use a 6-inch nonstick frying pan with an ovenproof handle. Don't forget the oven mitt or pot holder.

4 large eggs

3 tablespoons crumbled feta cheese

About 6 leaves fresh basil, minced or cut into very thin strips

Salt

Freshly ground black pepper

2 teaspoons extra-virgin olive oil

2 tablespoons minced scallion

One 7-inch zucchini (about 4 ounces), thinly sliced

½ teaspoon minced or crushed garlic

- *This makes 2 servings. If you are cooking for one, keep in mind that it tastes very good leftover at room temperature.*

▶ **YIELD: 2 SERVINGS**

Protein: 14 g / Saturated Fat: 4 g / Polyunsaturated Fat: 2 g / Monounsaturated Fat: 7 g / Dietary Fiber: 1 g / Calories: 204

1. Preheat the broiler to 500°F and move the oven rack to the highest position.

2. In a medium bowl, whisk the eggs until smooth, then stir in 1½ tablespoons of the feta, along with the basil, a pinch or two of salt, and a few grinds of pepper. Set aside.

3. Place the pan over medium heat and wait 1 minute. Add the oil and swirl to coat the pan. Add the scallion and zucchini, along with another pinch of salt. Sauté for about 2 to 3 minutes, or until the zucchini becomes light golden brown. At that point, stir in the garlic.

4. Pour in the egg mixture and let it sit still over the heat for about 30 seconds, then gently lift the edges with a spatula, and tilt the pan in all directions to let the loose egg move toward the edges. Allow it to sit for 5 minutes, until just about set. The top will still be wet.

5. Sprinkle on the remaining cheese, then transfer the pan to the broiler and broil for 2 to 3 minutes, or until the top is golden.

6. Using an oven mitt or pot holder, carefully remove the pan from the broiler, and let the frittata sit for about a minute to set. Loosen the edges with a spatula and transfer (sliding or flipping it) to a plate. Serve hot, warm, or at room temperature.

Whole-Grain French Toast

French toast is at its most delicious when the bread is completely soaked through and then cooked until crisp on the outside and creamy inside. The best way to accomplish this is to allow plenty of time for the pan to get hot and for the bread to absorb the custard. These can happen at the same time.

1 large egg
3 tablespoons low-fat milk
Pinch of salt
Pinch of cinnamon
Drop of vanilla extract
2 slices whole-grain bread*
Nonstick spray
1 teaspoon butter (optional)

▶ **YIELD: 1 SERVING**

Protein: 16 g / Saturated Fat: 2 g /
Polyunsaturated Fat: 1 g /
Monounsaturated Fat: 2 g /
Dietary Fiber: 8 g / Calories: 275

1. Place a large skillet or griddle over medium heat.
2. Break the egg into a pie pan and beat it with a fork until uniform and smooth.
3. Add the milk, salt, cinnamon, and vanilla, and stir until well blended.
4. Add the bread (the two slices should just fit, side by side), and let it sit in the custard for several minutes.
5. Turn the bread over and let it soak on the other side for another minute or so, tilting the pie pan to be sure all the liquid reaches the bread.
6. Lightly spray the hot skillet or griddle with nonstick spray, and, if you like, melt in a teaspoon or so of butter.
7. Fry the soaked bread for about 5 minutes (or until golden and toasty) on each side. Serve right away, plain, or with toppings of your choice.

*See Shopping Guide on page 264 for bread specifications.

MicroEggs

Scrambled eggs cooked in a microwave can be surprisingly good, and will spare you the extra steps of dealing with a frying pan, both before and after.

2 large eggs
2 tablespoons low-fat milk or water
Salt
Freshly ground black pepper

- *The milk can be whole or low-fat. If you use whole (and this tiny bit will not bust your diet), the results will be creamier.*

- To cook just one egg: *Divide everything by half. Use a 2-cup-capacity bowl and decrease the milk or water to 1 tablespoon. Cook for 20 seconds, stir, then continue cooking until the egg is set, about 20 seconds longer.*

▶ **YIELD: 1 SERVING**
Protein: 14 g / Saturated Fat: 4 g / Polyunsaturated Fat: 1 g / Monounsaturated Fat: 4 g / Dietary Fiber: 0 g / Calories: 166

1. In a 4-cup-capacity microwave-safe bowl, beat together the eggs, milk, a pinch of salt, and a grind or two of black pepper.
2. Cook on high for 40 seconds. Stir well, then resume cooking on high for 40 seconds longer, or until the egg is just set. (You might need an extra couple of seconds, but keep in mind that the egg will continue to cook a bit more after you take it out, and overcooking will cause it to become rubbery.) The surface will look wet, but there should be no moveable liquid remaining.
3. Enjoy directly in the bowl.

The Very Tall Sandwich— Permission to Raise the Roof

This is a strategy, rather than a recipe. You don't need to give up sandwiches in order to keep your weight down. In fact, you can make your sandwiches even larger than you otherwise would!

Begin with two slices of good whole-grain bread (see the specifications in the Shopping Guide, page 264) and spread one side with a little mayonnaise or a generous amount of Avocado "Butter" (page 187). Lavish the other side with some mustard or tomato-based salsa. Add a few slices of cheese or a palm-size serving of your Protein-of-Choice (pages 201–210). Then pile it high with vegetables: thin slices of cucumber; large, crisp leaves of romaine, spinach, or arugula; wheels of sweet red onion; sliced tomato; bell pepper (raw or roasted); grated carrot; and even perhaps some dill pickles (sliced the long way). Make the sandwich as tall as your mouth is high. Hold a plate under your chin when you take a bite, as pieces will tend to fall—and that's part of the fun.

Broiled Open-Face Cheddar Sandwich

Just because you're "on a diet" doesn't mean you can't enjoy some plain, old-fashioned melted cheese. Make that high-quality melted cheese, in this case. For once, instead of being limited to low-fat varieties, you get to choose any kind of deluxe Cheddar your heart may desire.

2 slices whole-grain bread*

Tomato-based salsa, mustard, or Sesame-Mustard Glaze (page 194)

1 ounce good Cheddar cheese (your favorite), grated

• *A toaster oven works best for this. If you don't have one, you can use the broiler.*

▶ **YIELD: 1 SERVING**
Protein: 15 g / Saturated Fat: 1 g /
Polyunsaturated Fat: 0 g /
Monounsaturated Fat: 1 g /
Dietary Fiber: 8 g / Calories: 234

1. Toast the bread to your liking.
2. Spoon on some salsa, mustard, or Sesame-Mustard Glaze.
3. Sprinkle the cheese over the top. Place the toast on the foil-lined tray of a toaster oven, and broil until the cheese is as melted as you want it. (Or place the toast on a small, foil-lined baking sheet and broil at 500°F.)

*See Shopping Guide on page 264 for bread specifications.

Ricotta Egg Salad

This little egg salad tastes wonderful when spread onto whole-grain crackers or thick cucumber slices.

1 large egg, hard-boiled, peeled and chopped fine

1 tablespoon finely minced parsley

1 tablespoon finely minced scallion

½ teaspoon grated lemon zest (optional)

1 tablespoon part-skim ricotta cheese

Salt

Freshly ground black pepper

Cayenne

• *This keeps for up to 5 days in a tightly covered container in the refrigerator.*

1. Combine the egg, parsley, scallion, and lemon zest in a small bowl and mix well.
2. Add the ricotta and continue to mix until well blended.
3. Season to taste with salt, pepper, and cayenne. Serve cold or at room temperature.

▶ **YIELD: 1 SERVING**
Protein: 8 g / Saturated Fat: 2 g /
Polyunsaturated Fat: 1 g /
Monounsaturated Fat: 2 g /
Dietary Fiber: 1 g / Calories: 100

Tofu "Egg" Salad

Surprisingly similar to the real thing! Serve this as you would regular egg salad—in a sandwich (on whole-grain bread or in a whole-wheat pita), or on a bed of greens, accompanied by olives, tomatoes, and fresh, raw vegetables.

6 ounces very firm tofu or nigari tofu

1 scallion, finely minced (include the green part)

3 tablespoons grated carrot

¼ cup finely minced celery

¼ cup finely minced red bell pepper

2 tablespoons toasted sunflower seeds

2 tablespoons mayonnaise

¼ teaspoon salt (or to taste)

Freshly ground black pepper

1. Cut the tofu into tiny dice and transfer to a medium-size bowl.
2. Add the remaining ingredients and mix gently.
3. Cover tightly and chill until cold.

- *This keeps for up to 5 days in a tightly covered container in the refrigerator.*

▶ **YIELD: 2 SERVINGS**

Protein: 8 g / Saturated Fat: 1 g / Polyunsaturated Fat: 6 g / Monounsaturated Fat: 2 g / Dietary Fiber: 2 g / Calories: 153

Nachos Lunch

One of the things people on weight-loss programs most often complain about missing is the sensation of biting into something crunchy. We've solved that by including this great little lunch option in the 21-Day Diet. It will make you feel like you're getting away with something—and, in fact, you are. Enjoy!

15 tortilla chips, as flat as possible

½ cup canned fat-free vegetarian refried beans

Tomato-based salsa

1 ounce low-fat Cheddar or Jack cheese, grated

- *A toaster oven works best for this, but you can also use a broiler.*

▶ **YIELD: 1 SERVING**

Protein: 17 g / Saturated Fat: 1 g /
Polyunsaturated Fat : < 1 g /
Monounsaturated Fat: 1 g /
Dietary Fiber: 9 g / Calories: 293

1. Preheat a toaster oven or conventional oven to 350°F. Line the toaster oven's baking tray (or a small baking sheet, if using the oven) with foil.

2. Place the tortilla chips on the tray in an even layer, not overlapping.

3. Use a teaspoon and your finger, if necessary, to dab small amounts of refried beans here and there onto the chips. You don't have to get them all.

4. Generously spoon as much salsa as you like on top of the beans.

5. Sprinkle the cheese over everything.

6. Place the tray in the oven until the cheese is melted and bubbling. This will take about 5 minutes. Keep your eye on it, so you'll be sure to take it out when it's done to your liking. Serve hot.

Portobello Pizzas

Portobello mushroom caps are ideal containers for vegetables and cheese. These fit perfectly onto toasted English muffins, and can thus be portable.

4 medium-size (4-inch) portobello mushrooms, caps
intact

Up to 1 tablespoon extra-virgin
olive oil

1 medium tomato

Half a medium yellow or
green bell pepper

1 handful fresh spinach
leaves, clean and dry

Dried thyme

Salt

Freshly ground black pepper

½ cup part-skim,
low-moisture mozzarella
cheese, shredded
(about 4 ounces)

Red pepper flakes (optional)

• *The fully cooked pizzas reheat
beautifully! Store in a tightly
covered container in the refrigerator, and bring to room temperature before reheating in a
300°F oven or a microwave.*

▶ YIELD: 2 SERVINGS (2 SMALL
PIZZAS APIECE)

Protein: 10 g / Saturated Fat: 3 g /
Polyunsaturated Fat: 1 g /
Monounsaturated Fat: 4 g /
Dietary Fiber: 2 g / Calories: 134

1. Remove the mushroom stems, and wipe the caps clean with a damp paper towel. Place a large, heavy skillet over medium heat for about 2 minutes. Add a little olive oil, wait about 30 seconds, then swirl to coat the pan. Place the mushrooms cap-side-down in the hot oil, and let them cook undisturbed for about 10 minutes. Turn them over and cook on the other side for 10 minutes, then flip them over one more time, to cook for about 5 to 10 more minutes on their cap side once again.

2. Meanwhile, core the tomato and gently squeeze out the seeds through the opening. Cut the tomato and bell pepper into very thin slices.

3. Shortly before serving, heat the broiler. While it is heating, place the mushrooms cap-side-down in an ovenproof glass or ceramic baking dish. Top each mushroom with a few spinach leaves; some slices of tomato and bell pepper; and pinches of dried thyme, salt, and pepper. Take your time covering the top with grated cheese, tucking it into every crevice and cavity, try-ing to cover everything (including the edges of the mushroom, so they won't burn under the broiler).

4. Broil until the cheese melts and is turning golden. Watch carefully, as this will take only 5 minutes or less. Serve hot, warm, or at room temperature, sprinkled with red pepper flakes if desired.

Avocado Waldorf

Easy and refreshing, this lunch salad looks its loveliest when made with a combination of green and red apples. Be sure the fruit is very crisp and fresh. Make this within an hour of eating, as it doesn't keep well.

3 medium apples (about 1 pound)

1 large stalk celery, minced

1 tablespoon raisins or dried cranberries

1 recipe Avocado-Yogurt Dressing (page 200)

¼ cup chopped, toasted walnuts

1. Cut the apples into bite-size chunks and transfer to a medium-size bowl.

2. Add the celery and raisins or cranberries, and toss.

3. Add the dressing and stir gently until everything is nicely coated.

4. Serve topped with the walnuts.

▶ **YIELD: 2 SERVINGS**

Protein: 5 g / Saturated Fat: 1 g /
Polyunsaturated Fat: 6 g /
Monounsaturated Fat: 2 g /
Dietary Fiber: 9 g / Calories: 245

Mediterranean-Style French Lentil Salad

Sweet and savory combine harmoniously in this colorful, fruity marinated salad. Streamline the preparation time by getting everything else ready while the lentils are cooking. The whole salad can be made up to two days ahead of time, but postpone adding the bell pepper and fresh herbs until shortly before serving.

1 cup dry French lentils

2 tablespoons extra-virgin olive oil

¼ teaspoon salt (or to taste)

1 orange, peeled and sectioned

½ teaspoon minced or crushed garlic

1½ tablespoons fresh lime juice

1½ tablespoons balsamic vinegar or cider vinegar

2 tablespoons very finely minced red onion

½ teaspoon each grated orange and lime zest (optional)

1 tablespoon dried currants

½ small carrot, shredded or finely minced

¼ cup minced bell pepper (a combination of red and yellow, if possible)

1 to 2 tablespoons minced fresh herbs, such as parsley, chives, and/or mint

1. Place the lentils in a pot and fill with enough water to cover them by 2 inches. Bring to a boil, then lower the heat to a simmer. Partially cover, and cook until the lentils are tender. (Check the water level and add more if necessary.) Cooking time should be around 20 to 30 minutes. Drain the lentils when they are done, and gently rinse in cold water. Drain again and place in a medium-large bowl.

2. Add the remaining ingredients except the bell pepper and fresh herbs, cover tightly, and chill at least 4 hours.

3. Add the bell pepper and herbs within an hour of serving. Serve cold or at room temperature.

- *French lentils are a small, round variety. They stay intact and slightly chewy after being cooked, and are thus a good choice for a salad. They need at least 4 hours to marinate after they are cooked, so plan ahead.*

- *If you are using the optional citrus zest(s), grate the fruit before sectioning it (orange), or juicing it (lime).*

▶ YIELD: 4 SERVINGS

Protein: 12 g / Saturated Fat: 1 g / Polyunsaturated Fat: 1 g / Monounsaturated Fat: 5 g / Dietary Fiber: 9 g / Calories: 245

Black Beans with Exotic Fruit

You can use canned lychees or pineapple (packed in juice) for this sparkling dish. You can also use fresh or frozen/defrosted mango. Don't worry if the fruit turns mushy and saucelike—that's actually preferable.

One 15-ounce can black beans, rinsed and drained (or 1¾ cups cooked black beans)

½ teaspoon minced or crushed garlic

2 tablespoons extra-virgin olive oil

½ teaspoon ground cumin

2 tablespoons very finely minced red onion

2 tablespoons fresh lemon juice or lime juice

⅓ cup finely chopped mango, lychee, or pineapple

¼ cup finely minced red bell pepper

¼ teaspoon salt (or to taste)

Cayenne

1. Combine the beans and garlic in a medium-size bowl.
2. Place the olive oil, cumin, and onion in a small bowl and microwave for about 20 seconds on high, then add this mixture to the beans and mix well.
3. Stir in the fruit juice, fruit, and bell pepper.
4. Add salt and cayenne to taste. Cover tightly and refrigerate until serving.

- This keeps for about 5 days in a tightly covered container in the refrigerator.

- It tastes good freshly made, but is even better as it sits around (best on the second or third day), as this waiting period allows the beans to absorb the other flavors.

▶ **YIELD: 3 SERVINGS**
Protein: 9 g / Saturated Fat: 1 g / Polyunsaturated Fat: 1 g / Monounsaturated Fat: 7 g / Dietary Fiber: 9 g / Calories: 231

Quick Marinated White Beans

You can throw this together in minutes flat. It keeps well for about 5 days (stored in a tightly covered container in the refrigerator), and although the flavor does improve as it marinates, it tastes very good right out of the gate.

One 15-ounce can white navy beans or pea beans, rinsed and drained (or 1¾ cups cooked white beans)

2 tablespoons extra-virgin olive oil

1 tablespoon red wine vinegar (or more)

¼ teaspoon salt (or to taste)

½ teaspoon minced or crushed garlic

½ teaspoon dried basil (or 1 tablespoon minced fresh basil, if available)

¼ teaspoon dried oregano

Freshly ground black pepper

Optional additions:

2 tablespoons minced fresh parsley

2 tablespoons finely minced carrot

2 tablespoons finely minced celery

1. Combine everything in a medium-size bowl.
2. Taste to see if it needs more salt or vinegar.
3. Cover tightly and refrigerate until serving time.

▶ **YIELD: 3 SERVINGS**

Protein: 9 g / Saturated Fat: 1 g /
Polyunsaturated Fat: 1 g /
Monounsaturated Fat: 7 g /
Dietary Fiber: 11 g / Calories: 232

Pickled Red Onions

Red onions have a secret talent: They turn a beautiful, bright shade of purplish-pink when doused with hot water and then marinated, and in this pickled state, they stay crunchy and delicious seemingly forever.

3 medium-size red onions
(about 1 pound)
4 cups boiling water

Marinade:

½ cup cider vinegar
½ cup water
3 tablespoons sugar or
light-colored honey
½ teaspoon salt
Freshly ground black pepper
(a few grinds)

- *Serve Pickled Red Onions in every imaginable context: next to or over hot or cold bean and grain dishes, with (or in) salads or sandwiches, on toast or crackers, with hors d'oeuvres— you name it.*

- *These keep for months in a tightly covered container in the refrigerator.*

▶ YIELD: ABOUT 3½ CUPS
Protein: < 1 g / Saturated Fat: 0 g /
Polyunsaturated Fat: 0 g /
Monounsaturated Fat: 0 g /
Dietary Fiber: < 1 g / Calories: 19

1. Peel the onions and slice them as thin as you possibly can with a very sharp knife. Transfer them to a medium-size bowl.
2. Pour the boiling water into the bowl, and let the onions soak for 5 minutes. Drain thoroughly in a colander.
3. While the onions sit in the colander, combine the marinade ingredients in the same bowl, and mix well. Stir in the onions, and let them sit in the marinade for about 10 minutes.
4. Transfer the onions with all the liquid to a jar with a tight-fitting lid, and chill until very cold.

Marinated Cucumbers

The clean, cool taste of this very pure dish provides a good contrast to hot entrées with more complex flavors. You have the option of making this plain, or of spicing it up, Thai-style, with hot chilis and fresh cilantro.

¼ cup cider vinegar

2 teaspoons sugar

¼ teaspoon salt (or to taste)

2 medium-size cucumbers
(about 8 inches long)

½ cup very finely minced
red onion

Optional additions:

1 small red or green serrano
chili, seeded and cut into
very thin, small strips

2 to 3 tablespoons minced
fresh cilantro

- *If you decide to add the chilis, be very careful handling them, as the heat can permeate everything they touch (including your hands, and therefore, possibly, your eyes). So wash your hands and the cutting surface when you are finished preparing it.*

- *Marinated Cucumbers keep for several weeks in a tightly covered container in the refrigerator, and they improve with age.*

1. Combine the vinegar, sugar, and salt in a medium-size bowl.
2. Peel and seed the cucumbers. (It's easiest to halve them lengthwise and scrape out the seeds with a spoon.) Cut them into quarters lengthwise, then into very thin slices.
3. Add the cucumbers, onion, and chilis and cilantro, if using, to the vinegar mixture and stir to combine.
4. Transfer to a jar with a lid, cover tightly, and marinate in the refrigerator for at least 4 hours and up to several weeks.

▶ YIELD: 6 ¼-CUP SERVINGS
Protein: 1 g / Saturated Fat: 0 g /
Polyunsaturated Fat: 0 g /
Monounsaturated Fat: 0 g /
Dietary Fiber: 1 g / Calories: 28

Taboo-less Tabouleh

Here's a greened-up version of the classic bulgur wheat salad, making it more herb-and vegetable-centric. The best tool for making this dish is a food processor that has a small bowl (or a mini food processor), so you can mince the parsley, mint, and scallions into a fine, feathery state with the push of a button.

½ cup dry bulgur

½ cup boiling water

2 scallions, tips trimmed

½ cup (packed measure) fresh parsley

10 medium-size fresh mint leaves

½ teaspoon minced or crushed garlic

¼ teaspoon salt (or to taste)

2 tablespoons extra-virgin olive oil

2 tablespoons fresh lemon juice

1 small cucumber, seeded and finely minced (peeling optional)

Half a small bell pepper (a yellow or orange one, if possible), finely minced

Freshly ground black pepper

1 medium-size ripe tomato, cut into tiny dice

1. Combine the bulgur and boiling water in a medium-size bowl, and cover the bowl with a plate. Let stand for 20 minutes.
2. Cut the scallions into large pieces (including the green parts) and place in the small bowl of a food processor (or in a mini food processor) with the parsley and mint, and chop until tiny. (Or, if you don't have a food processor, use a sharp knife to do this job.)
3. Add the garlic, salt, half the olive oil, and half the lemon juice to the bulgur and stir well.
4. Stir in the minced herbs and all the other ingredients, including the remaining olive oil and lemon juice. Cover tightly and refrigerate until serving time.

- *Tabouleh will keep for up to a week if stored in a tightly covered container in the refrigerator. It tastes best after it has had a chance to sit for at least an hour, so the flavors can develop.*

▶ YIELD: 2 MAIN-DISH SERVINGS

Protein: 8 g / Saturated Fat: 2 g / Polyunsaturated Fat: 2 g / Monounsaturated Fat: 10 g / Dietary Fiber: 13 g / Calories: 347

SOUPS

Ten-Minute Tomato Soup

Roasted Garlic Paste makes this soup taste really wonderful, and the "10-minute" promise of the recipe title assumes you have some on hand. Realizing that this is not entirely fair, and that you may not yet be in the habit of keeping some of this great ingredient around at all times, we offer you a choice of substituting fresh garlic cooked briefly in olive oil (see first note below). The soup will be good either way.

One 28-ounce can tomatoes (whole or crushed)

1 tablespoon Roasted Garlic Paste (page 185)—or see note below

A dozen leaves fresh basil—or 1 tablespoon dried basil

Pinch of salt (optional)

Freshly ground black pepper

Cayenne or red pepper flakes

1 tablespoon extra-virgin olive oil

1. Combine the tomatoes, Roasted Garlic Paste or sautéed garlic, and basil in a blender or food processor, and puree to your desired texture.

2. Transfer to a pot and place over medium heat. Bring to a boil, lower the heat to a simmer, and cook, partially covered, for 5 minutes or a little longer.

3. Season to taste and drizzle in the extra-virgin olive oil. Serve hot.

- *If you don't have Roasted Garlic Paste on hand, use 2 teaspoons minced or crushed fresh garlic, sautéed lightly (10 to 20 seconds) in 1 tablespoon extra-virgin olive oil.*

- *This keeps for up to a week if stored in a tightly covered container in the refrigerator.*

▶ YIELD: 3 SERVINGS (A GENEROUS ¾ CUP PER SERVING)

Protein: 3 g / Saturated Fat: 1 g / Polyunsaturated Fat: 1 g / Monounsaturated Fat: 4 g / Dietary Fiber: 3 g / Calories: 112

Ethereal Broccoli Soup

Both this recipe and its Delicate Spinach counterpart (opposite page) are practically instant soups! Pureeing vegetables into soup is one of the easiest and most delightful ways to go green(er) with your diet. These two recipes are terrific hunger-busters that will fill you up just the right amount. And if they don't do the trick on the first go-round, just help yourself to more. We're happy to report that these soups are an "unlimited" item on the 21-Day Diet!

2 cups vegetable broth

2 cups chopped broccoli, fresh or frozen (6 to 10 ounces)

Salt (optional)

Freshly ground black pepper (optional)

- *There are several good vegetable broths available commercially. This recipe was tested with Imagine Organic Vegetable Broth, available in most grocery stores, stored unrefrigerated in 1-quart boxes (similar to soy milk packaging).*

- *You can make this soup with fresh or frozen broccoli. If using frozen, you don't need to defrost it ahead of time.*

- *This soup will keep for up to 5 days if stored in a tightly covered container in the refrigerator.*

▶ **YIELD: 2 SERVINGS**
Protein: 5 g / Saturated Fat: 0 g / Polyunsaturated Fat: 0 g / Monounsaturated Fat: < 1 g / Dietary Fiber: 6 g / Calories: 77

1. Pour the broth into a medium-size saucepan and bring to a boil.
2. Add the broccoli, partially cover, and cook over medium heat for 3 minutes if the broccoli is fresh, or for 5 minutes if it's frozen.
3. Remove from heat and let stand, uncovered, for 5 minutes.
4. Transfer to a blender and puree to your desired texture. (Or you can use an immersion blender to puree the soup directly in the pot.)
5. Season to taste with salt and pepper. Serve hot.

Delicate Spinach Soup

There are several good vegetable broths available commercially. This recipe was tested with Imagine Organic Vegetable Broth, available in most grocery stores, stored unrefrigerated in 1-quart boxes (similar to soy milk packaging).

2 cups vegetable broth

2 cups (firmly packed) fresh spinach leaves, or 1 (10 ounce) package frozen spinach

Salt (optional)

Freshly ground black pepper (optional)

Freshly grated nutmeg

- *You can make this with fresh or frozen spinach. If using frozen, you don't need to defrost it ahead of time.*

- *This will keep for up to 5 days if stored in a tightly covered container in the refrigerator.*

▶ **YIELD: 2 SERVINGS**

Protein: 7 g / Saturated Fat: < 1 g / Polyunsaturated Fat: 0 g / Monounsaturated Fat: 0 g / Dietary Fiber: 6 g / Calories: 82

1. Pour the broth into a medium-size saucepan and bring to a boil.

2. Add the spinach, partially cover, and cook over medium heat for 3 minutes (if the spinach is fresh) or for 5 minutes (if it's frozen).

3. Remove from heat and let stand, uncovered, for 5 minutes.

4. Transfer to a blender and puree to your desired texture. (Or you can use an immersion blender to puree the soup directly in the pot.)

5. Season to taste with salt, pepper, and nutmeg. Serve hot.

Miso Soup with Tofu and Scallions

Rich in enzymes that aid digestion, miso is a salty, deeply flavored paste made from aged fermented soybeans and grains. There are many varieties of miso (determined by variations in the soybeans, the type of grain used, length of fermentation, etc.) and they are often referred to by their color (red, yellow, brown, white, etc.). Because it is already fermented and aged, miso keeps indefinitely on your pantry shelf and, once opened, can be stored for several months in the refrigerator. You can buy it at Japanese and Asian markets, and also in many grocery stores (especially natural-food groceries). The best type of miso to use for this soup is shiro or "mellow white," but any type will work.

A single portion of miso soup can be put together—and ready to serve—in roughly the amount of time it takes to brew a cup of tea. Try transferring the soup to a wide-neck thermos and take it to work with you. If you are too hurried to make even this simple recipe—or you don't have the ingredients on hand—there are some very good brands of instant miso soup powder available. They come in single-serving packets, and all you need to do is add hot water and stir. Consider keeping a stash at work, for spontaneous nourishment.

1 tablespoon miso
1 cup boiling water
1 to 2 tablespoons diced tofu
(any kind) (tiny pieces)
1 tablespoon very finely
minced scallion

▶ YIELD: 1 SERVING

Protein: 3 g / Saturated Fat: 0 g /
Polyunsaturated Fat: 1 g /
Monounsaturated Fat: 0 g /
Dietary Fiber: 1 g / Calories: 41

1. Place the miso in a generously sized single-serving bowl, and pour in about ⅓ of the boiling water. Mash and stir until the mixture becomes smooth.
2. Add the remaining hot water, along with the tofu and scallion.
3. Serve right away.

Variations

Miso soup is delicious plain, sipped like a hot beverage. You can also make it into a heartier meal by adding any or all of the following:

- A few spoonfuls of cooked grains (wild rice or barley is especially nice)
- A poached egg
- A handful of daikon sprouts or radish sprouts
- Wakame (a sea vegetable that comes dried)—soaked in tap water for 15 minutes, or until tender
- A few small spinach leaves

Vegetable Broth
and Its Many Possibilities

A full-flavored broth with a few accents can be an incredibly useful and soothing addition to any eating plan. When consumed at the beginning of a meal, broth calms us down and not only takes the edge off our appetite—it whets it, warming up (literally and poetically) our taste buds for the food to follow.

Once upon a time, "vegetable broth" meant either a very salty and thin-flavored (okay, pathetic) bouillon cube dissolved in boiling water, or an unpredictable potful of scraps and water simmered on your stove. These days, however, there are several very good vegetable broths available commercially. Several of them are so good, in fact, that you can pretty much enjoy them straight from the box—plain, or with just a few accoutrements added. (And we literally mean "box," as these broths are available in most grocery stores, stored unrefrigerated in 1-quart boxes, similar to those used for soy milk.) Our favorite brand is Imagine Organic Vegetable Broth, but there are others to choose from, including Swanson and Pacific. Taste a few and find your own favorite.

Here are some ideas for augmenting vegetable broth in single-serving proportions (except for the one made with egg, which serves two). All of these will keep up to a week in a tightly covered container in the refrigerator.

Vegetable Broth with Mushrooms and Barley

1 cup vegetable broth

1 medium-size mushroom, thinly sliced

1 tablespoon cooked barley (page 55)

1 tablespoon finely minced scallion

▶ YIELD: 1 SERVING

Protein: 2 g / Saturated Fat: 0 g / Polyunsaturated Fat: 0 g / Monounsaturated Fat: 0 g / Dietary Fiber: 2 g / Calories: 54

1. Place the broth into a bowl, and heat in the microwave on high for 1½ minutes, or until steaming hot—or heat in a small saucepan on the stovetop until just about boiling.
2. Add the sliced mushroom to the hot broth. It will cook upon contact.
3. Stir in the barley and scallion, and serve hot.

Vegetable Broth with Corn

1 cup vegetable broth

2 tablespoons fresh or frozen corn kernels, cooked

1 tablespoon finely minced scallion

▶ YIELD: 1 SERVING

Protein: 2 g / Saturated Fat: 0 g / Polyunsaturated Fat: 0 g / Monounsaturated Fat: 0 g / Dietary Fiber: 2 g / Calories: 60

1. Place the broth in a bowl, and heat in the microwave on high for 1½ minutes, or until steaming hot—or heat in a small saucepan on the stovetop until just about boiling.
2. Stir in the corn and scallion. Serve hot.

Vegetable Broth with Egg

This is similar to the egg-drop soup made in Chinese restaurants.

2 cups vegetable broth

1 large egg, beaten

1 tablespoon finely minced scallion

▶ YIELD: 2 SERVINGS

Protein: 4 g / Saturated Fat: 1 g / Polyunsaturated Fat: 0 g / Monounsaturated Fat: 1 g / Dietary Fiber: 1 g / Calories: 73

1. Place the broth in a medium-small saucepan on the stovetop, and heat until just about boiling.
2. Turn off the heat, and pour in the beaten egg. Stir for about 30 seconds, as the egg fluffs up and cooks from the heat of the broth.
3. Add the scallion, and serve hot.

Vegetable Broth with Vermicelli and Peas

1 cup vegetable broth

2 tablespoons frozen peas

2 tablespoons cooked
vermicelli noodles

▶ YIELD: 1 SERVING

Protein: 3 g / Saturated Fat: 0 g /
Polyunsaturated Fat: 0 g /
Monounsaturated Fat: 0 g /
Dietary Fiber: 2 g / Calories: 69

1. Place the broth and peas in a bowl, and heat in the microwave on high for 1½ to 2 minutes, or until steaming hot—or heat in a small saucepan on the stovetop until the broth is just about boiling and the peas are cooked.
2. Add the vermicelli. Serve hot.

Vegetable Broth with White Beans

You can use freshly cooked white beans or the canned variety. If using canned, rinse and drain the beans well before adding to the soup.

1 cup vegetable broth

2 tablespoons cooked white
beans

▶ YIELD: 1 SERVING

Protein: 3 g / Saturated Fat: 0 g /
Polyunsaturated Fat: 0 g /
Monounsaturated Fat: 0 g /
Dietary Fiber: 3 g / Calories: 57

1. Place the broth in a bowl, and heat in the microwave on high for 1½ minutes, or until steaming hot—or heat in a small saucepan on the stovetop until just about boiling.
2. Spoon in the beans. Serve hot.

Vegetable Broth with Wheat Berries or Wild Rice

1 cup vegetable broth

2 tablespoons cooked
wheat berries or wild rice
(pages 54–56)

▶ YIELD: 1 SERVING

Protein: 2 g / Saturated Fat: 0 g /
Polyunsaturated Fat: 0 g /
Monounsaturated Fat: 0 g /
Dietary Fiber: 1 g / Calories: 56

1. Place the broth in a bowl, and heat in the microwave on high for 1½ minutes, or until steaming hot—or heat in a small saucepan on the stovetop until just about boiling.
2. Spoon in the grains. Serve hot.

Gazpacho

The famous cold tomato-based soup, reduced to its delicious essence! Although thickened with vegetables—rather than with the traditional bread used by Spanish cooks—this light gazpacho is still thin enough to drink, but also has enough heft to make you feel utterly satisfied.

1 pound very ripe tomatoes, cored and cut into chunks—or 1 (28-ounce) can tomatoes (whole or crushed)

1½ cups cucumber chunks (peeled and seeded)

½ cup chopped bell pepper

A handful of parsley

½ teaspoon minced or crushed garlic

¼ teaspoon ground cumin

½ teaspoon salt

1 teaspoon red wine vinegar

1 teaspoon light-colored honey

2 teaspoons fresh lemon juice

1 tablespoon extra-virgin olive oil

Cayenne

1. Place the tomatoes in a blender or food processor with all the remaining ingredients except the cayenne.
2. Puree to your desired texture.
3. Transfer to a container with a tight-fitting lid, and add cayenne to taste. Cover and chill for at least 4 hours. Serve cold.

- *Make this at least 4 hours ahead of time, as it needs to chill.*
- *This keeps for a week or longer if refrigerated in a tightly covered container.*

▶ **YIELD: 4 SERVINGS**
Protein: 2 g / Saturated Fat: < 1 g / Polyunsaturated Fat: 0 g / Monounsaturated Fat: 3 g / Dietary Fiber: 2 g / Calories: 69

SNACKS

Super Trail Mix

Sometimes we need to be able to nibble on a snack that is light and airy as well as satisfying. This way we can stretch out the grazing, and make it last longer without blowing our healthy eating plan. Other times, though, we need concentrated mid-afternoon fortification that we can enjoy in just a few bites before moving on to the next activity. Here are two versions of the 21-Day Diet's signature snack, Super Trail Mix: One is a potent mix of nuts and dried fruit with less volume and more intensity. The other is literally a fluffier combination that also includes puffed whole-grain cereal, to extend the experience into more of a contained munch-fest. Take your pick! The recipes appear on the following page.

> NOTE: A good way to control Super Trail Mix portion size is to measure single servings into small resealable plastic bags as soon as it's made. Store the bags in the refrigerator, and just pull them out, one at a time, as needed.

Super Trail Mix One

1 cup mixed nuts (walnuts, pecans, cashews, almonds, peanuts)

¼ cup raisins

¼ cup dried cranberries

Combine everything, and store in a resealable plastic bag (or four resealable single-serving bags) in the refrigerator.

▶ YIELD: 4 SERVINGS (6 TABLE-SPOONS PER SERVING)

Protein: 6 g / Saturated Fat: 1 g / Polyunsaturated Fat: 6 g / Monounsaturated Fat: 1 g / Dietary Fiber: 4 g / Calories: 240

Super Trail Mix Two

The best puffed cereals to use for this lighter mixture are Kashi 7 Whole Grain Puffs or Nature's Path Organic Corn Puffs cereal. A combination of the two is very nice.

1 cup mixed nuts (walnuts, pecans, cashews, almonds, peanuts)

¼ cup raisins

¼ cup dried cranberries

3½ cups unsweetened whole-grain puffed cereal

Combine everything, and store in a resealable plastic bag (or five resealable single-serving bags) in the refrigerator.

▶ YIELD: 5 SERVINGS (1 CUP PER SERVING)

Protein: 6 g / Saturated Fat: 1 g / Polyunsaturated Fat: 5 g / Monounsaturated Fat: 1 g / Dietary Fiber: 4 g / Calories: 241

Baked Vanilla-Cinnamon-Coated Nuts

A sweet egg coating baked onto nuts practically makes them into cookies. This is a heavenly portable snack, and it's also great for entertaining.

Nonstick spray for the baking sheet

2 large eggs

1 teaspoon pure vanilla extract

½ teaspoon cinnamon (rounded measure)

½ teaspoon salt (rounded measure)

⅓ cup granulated sugar (or more)

5 cups raw, unsalted nuts in large pieces (any combination of whole almonds, cashews, and/or walnut or pecan halves)

- *Store these in a tightly closed jar for several weeks in the refrigerator, or for several months in the freezer.*

- *One batch makes a good twenty servings (and they are very good)!*

▶ **YIELD: 20 SERVINGS (1 HEAPING ¼ CUP—10 TO 12 PIECES—PER SERVING)**

Protein: 7 g / Saturated Fat: 2 g / Polyunsaturated Fat: 8 g / Monounsaturated Fat: 7 g / Dietary Fiber: 3 g / Calories: 208

1. Preheat the oven to 300°F. Generously spray a baking sheet with nonstick spray.

2. Break the eggs into a large bowl and beat well with a fork or whisk. Add the vanilla, cinnamon, salt, and ⅓ cup sugar, and beat until blended.

3. Add the nuts and stir until they are thoroughly moistened. Let stand 5 minutes.

4. Transfer the nuts, plus any remaining liquid, to the prepared baking sheet, and push together into a single layer, so the nuts are touching, but not piled vertically. (It should be one large, flat mass.)

5. Bake on the center rack of the oven for 15 minutes, then use a spatula to scrape the nuts and their coating from the bottom of the baking sheet, and rearrange everything, so nothing is sticking and the nuts get moved around a bit. This helps them cook evenly.

6. Bake another 15 minutes, then remove from the oven. If your taste runs sweet, you can sprinkle the nuts with 1 to 2 teaspoons additional sugar while they are still hot and on the baking sheet. Let the nuts cool completely on the baking sheet, then transfer them to clean jars with tight-fitting lids for storage. (You can also just transfer them to bowls for instant eating.)

Baked Cajun-Style Savory-Coated Nuts

A spicy coating baked onto these nuts makes them crisp and highly flavorful. They make a very fulfilling portable snack, and are perfect for entertaining, too.

Nonstick spray for the baking sheet

2 large eggs

1 tablespoon soy sauce

1 tablespoon Worcestershire sauce (optional)

½ teaspoon salt

4 teaspoons ground cumin

1 teaspoon dried thyme

¼ teaspoon cayenne

4 cups raw, unsalted nuts in large pieces (any combination of whole almonds, cashews, and/or walnut or pecan halves)

Up to 2 tablespoons fresh lemon or lime juice (optional)

- *Store the nuts in a tightly closed jar for several weeks in the refrigerator—or for several months in the freezer.*

- *One batch makes sixteen servings!*

▶ YIELD: 16 SERVINGS (1 HEAP-ING ¼ CUP—10 TO 12 PIECES—PER SERVING)

Protein: 7 g / Saturated Fat: 2 g / Polyunsaturated Fat: 8 g / Monounsaturated Fat: 7 g / Dietary Fiber: 3 g / Calories: 200

1. Preheat the oven to 300°F. Generously spray a baking sheet with nonstick spray.
2. Break the eggs into a large bowl and beat well with a fork or whisk. Add the soy sauce, Worcestershire sauce, if using, salt, cumin, thyme, and cayenne, and beat until blended.
3. Add the nuts and stir until they are thoroughly moistened. Let stand 5 minutes.
4. Transfer the nuts, plus any remaining liquid, to the prepared baking sheet, and push together into a single layer, so the nuts are touching, but not piled vertically. (It should be one large, flat mass.) If you like a tart flavor, sprinkle the top with up to 2 tablespoons fresh lemon or lime juice.
5. Bake on the center rack of the oven for 15 minutes, then use a spatula to scrape the nuts and their coating from the bottom of the baking sheet, and rearrange everything, so nothing is sticking and the nuts get moved around a bit. This helps them cook evenly.
6. Bake another 15 minutes, then remove the baking sheet from the oven. Let the nuts cool completely on the baking sheet, then transfer them to clean jars with tight-fitting lids for storage. (You can also just transfer them to bowls for instant eating.)

Carrot-Almond-Oat Gems

Soft and chewy—and brimming with grated carrot and almonds—these dense nuggets are deeply satisfying and make a great portable breakfast or snack. They are packed with fiber and vitamins, and will fill you up while also taking care of your sweet tooth.

Nonstick spray for the pan
2 cups whole almonds
¼ cup rolled oats
3 to 4 tablespoons sugar
½ teaspoon salt
(scant measure)
1½ cups (packed) finely
shredded carrot
(about ½ pound)
1 to 2 teaspoons grated lemon
zest
1 teaspoon vanilla extract
⅛ teaspoon almond extract

- This recipe is truly quick and easy if you use a food processor for grinding the almonds and grating the carrots. If you don't have a food processor, you can do step 2 in a blender, and grate the carrots by hand.

- A mild honey or pure maple syrup can replace the sugar. If using either of these, add it with the grated carrot in step 3.

▶ YIELD: ABOUT 1 DOZEN
PIECES

Protein: 6 g / Saturated Fat: 1 g /
Polyunsaturated Fat: 3 g /
Monounsaturated Fat: 8 g /
Dietary Fiber: 3 g / Calories: 168

1. Preheat the oven to 350°F. Lightly spray an 8-inch round cake pan with nonstick spray.

2. Place 1½ cups of the almonds in a food processor fitted with a steel blade. Add the oats, sugar, and salt, and process with a few long pulses until they combine to become a powder. Transfer this to a medium-size bowl. Finely chop the remaining ½ cup of the almonds and stir these in.

3. Using the fine-grating attachment of the food processor, grate the carrot(s). Add this to the almond mixture, along with lemon zest and extracts, and mix with a fork until thoroughly combined.

4. Transfer the batter to the center of the prepared pan, and shape it into a circle about 1 inch high and 6½ inches in diameter. Bake on the center rack of the oven for 30 minutes or until dry on top.

5. Remove the pan from the oven, and cut the baked mixture into pieces while still hot. (You get to choose the size and shape of the pieces. Cutting a dozen wedge-shaped "gems" works well.) Cool in the pan for about 20 minutes, then transfer to a rack to cool for at least 15 minutes longer. Store in a tightly covered container in the refrigerator, and serve cold or at room temperature.

Date-Peanut–Flax Seed No-Bake Nuggets

Here is one terrific vehicle for flax seeds, which can't really be effectively consumed on their own.

1⅓ cups (packed) pitted dates (about ½ pound)

½ cup flax seeds

½ cup peanuts

½ cup dried cranberries (optional)

½ to ¾ cup peanut butter (salted or not)

1 to 2 tablespoons flaxseed oil (optional)

½ cup shredded unsweetened coconut (optional)

- Use a high-quality "natural" peanut butter for best results.

- Purchase flax seed in bulk at natural-food stores, and store in a cool, dark place.

- These will keep for weeks or even months (if you don't eat them sooner) when stored in a tightly covered container in the refrigerator or freezer.

▶ YIELD: ABOUT 2 DOZEN NUGGETS

Protein: 3 g / Saturated Fat: 2 g /
Polyunsaturated Fat: 2 g /
Monounsaturated Fat: 2 g /
Dietary Fiber: 2 g / Calories: 92

1. Place the dates in a medium-size bowl. Mash them with a spoon if they are soft and sticky. If you're using dates that are drier or in rolled form, just break them into smaller pieces with your fingers or cut them with scissors, then put them in the bowl and push them together with a spoon.

2. Grind the flax seeds—and then the peanuts—to a fine meal in an electric spice grinder or a blender. (Process with a few short buzzes, rather than long pulses, to be sure they don't get too oily and turn into paste.) Add them to the dates, using a fork or your fingers to rub everything together. Mix in the dried cranberries as you go.

3. Add the peanut butter, mixing and mashing it in with a spoon or your hands. You can also add some flaxseed oil at this point, to help everything hold together (and for added nutrition).

4. Use your hands, or two spoons, to scoop up heaping teaspoons of the mixture, and shape each piece into a tight little ball (about 1 inch in diameter). Roll each ball in the coconut, if desired. Place the nuggets in a shallow plastic container with a tight-fitting lid, and refrigerate or freeze as soon as you're done. Eat at room temperature or cold—or even frozen, if you like!

Pistachio-Currant Halvah No-Bake Nuggets

So satisfying and good for you, these will work their way into the heart of your busy lifestyle as a grabbed breakfast on the run, or an afternoon pick-me-up snack.

1 cup sesame tahini

2 tablespoons light-colored honey

½ teaspoon salt (scant measure)

⅔ cup dried currants

⅔ cup minced or ground pistachio nuts, lightly toasted

⅓ cup sesame seeds (hulled or unhulled)

- *These keep for weeks or even months if stored in a tightly covered container in the refrigerator or freezer.*

▶ **YIELD: 2 DOZEN NUGGETS**

Protein: 3 g / Saturated Fat: 1 g /
Polyunsaturated Fat: 4 g /
Monounsaturated Fat: 4 g /
Dietary Fiber: 2 g / Calories: 115

1. Combine the tahini, honey, and salt in a medium-size bowl, and use a fork or the back of a spoon to mix and/or mash them together until reasonably well blended.

2. Add the currants and pistachio nuts, mashing them in as best you can. It will be a little stiff.

3. Place the sesame seeds on a plate. Use your hands (wetting them, if necessary) to make the tahini mixture into 1-inch balls, then roll each ball in the sesame seeds until thoroughly coated.

4. Place the coated nuggets in a shallow plastic container with a tight-fitting lid, and store in the refrigerator or freezer. Eat them cold or at room temperature—or even frozen, if you like!

SMOOTHIES AND SHAKES

The basic smoothie method is very low-tech: Throw all the ingredients into a blender and push the button. If you have access to a blender and a refrigerator at work, it's a lovely idea to keep smoothie ingredients on hand and whip up any of these recipes for a good midafternoon refreshment.

Smoothies keep for several days if stored in a tightly covered container in the refrigerator, but they do tend to separate, so shake well before serving.

Whey protein powder (an optional addition) is a lactose-free nutritional supplement that comes in large cans in natural-food groceries, vitamin shops, and health-food stores. It lasts for a long time without refrigeration, and can add a nice hit of stealth protein to these smoothies.

It is okay to use frozen fruit for any of these recipes. You don't need to defrost it first, but do chop it into small pieces with a very sharp knife, so the smoothie will blend well.

Cantaloupe-Peach Smoothie

You can also make this with just cantaloupe—or with only peaches. It works well all three ways.

½ cup orange juice

½ cup nonfat vanilla yogurt*

2 tablespoons fresh lemon juice

1 cup cantaloupe chunks

1 cup sliced peaches

5 to 6 ice cubes

1 tablespoon unsweetened vanilla-flavored whey protein powder (optional)

1 tablespoon real maple syrup or light-colored honey—or non-caloric sweetener to taste (optional)

Place everything in a blender and puree to desired consistency. Serve cold. (If you refrigerate the smoothie overnight, it will thicken slightly and might separate. So stir or shake before serving.)

▶ **YIELD: 2 SERVINGS**
Protein: 5 g / Saturated Fat: < 1 g / Polyunsaturated Fat: < 1 g / Monounsaturated Fat: < 1 g / Dietary Fiber: < 1 g / Calories: 147

Honeydew Smoothie

½ cup orange juice

½ cup nonfat vanilla yogurt*

¼ cup fresh lemon juice

2 to 3 cups honeydew chunks

5 to 6 ice cubes

A handful of fresh mint leaves (optional)

1 tablespoon unsweetened vanilla-flavored whey protein powder (optional)

1 tablespoon real maple syrup or light-colored honey—or non-caloric sweetener to taste (optional)

Place everything in a blender and puree to desired consistency. Serve cold. (If you refrigerate the smoothie overnight, it will thicken slightly and might separate. So stir or shake before serving.)

▶ **YIELD: 2 SERVINGS**
Protein: 5 g / Saturated Fat: < 1 g / Polyunsaturated Fat: < 1 g / Monounsaturated Fat: < 1 g / Dietary Fiber: 2 g / Calories: 149

*See Shopping Guide (page 267) for yogurt specifications.

Strawberry-Banana Smoothie

This is especially good when made with frozen strawberries. If you're using the individually frozen kind, you don't need to defrost them first, but do chop them into small pieces with a very sharp knife, so they will blend in well. (They don't have to blend in completely— a little texture is nice.)

½ cup orange juice

½ cup nonfat vanilla yogurt*

1 to 2 tablespoons fresh lemon juice

Half a medium-size ripe banana (about ½ cup, sliced)

8 to 10 large strawberries

5 to 6 ice cubes

1 tablespoon unsweetened vanilla-flavored whey protein powder (optional)

1 tablespoon real maple syrup or light-colored honey—or non-caloric sweetener to taste (optional)

Place everything in a blender and puree to desired consistency. Serve cold. (If you refrigerate the smoothie overnight, it will thicken slightly and might separate. So stir or shake before serving.)

▶ YIELD: 2 SERVINGS

Protein: 4 g / Saturated Fat: < 1 g / Polyunsaturated Fat: < 1 g / Monounsaturated Fat: < 1 g / Dietary Fiber: 3 g / Calories: 140

Chocolate-Banana Shake

Okay, so sweetened cocoa powder is not the most enlightened ingredient in the world, but it is well worth the satisfaction you get with this quick and delightful fix. For an even frothier and frostier effect, use a frozen banana. (This presupposes you have remembered to freeze one.)

1 cup 1% low-fat milk

½ medium-size ripe banana

1 to 2 tablespoons sweetened cocoa powder

3 to 4 ice cubes (or about ½ cup crushed ice)

Combine everything in a blender. Cover and puree to desired consistency. Pour into a tall glass and enjoy!

▶ YIELD: 1 SERVING

Protein: 9 g / Saturated Fat: 2 g / Polyunsaturated Fat: 0 g / Monounsaturated Fat: 1 g / Dietary Fiber: 3 g / Calories: 238

*See Shopping Guide (page 267) for yogurt specifications.

SAUCES, SALAD DRESSINGS, AND DIPS

Roasted Garlic Paste

A wonderful basic condiment on its own, or an ingredient for other things, Roasted Garlic Paste has a surprisingly mild and friendly flavor. The sharpness that we normally expect is dramatically softened through the roasting process, and the result is pungent in a very positive sense.

3 tablespoons extra-virgin olive oil (or more)

3 medium heads garlic (about 3 ounces each)

- *This recipe is very easily multiplied. Get into the habit of making multiple batches and keep this magical stuff on hand as a staple.*

- *This keeps well for a week or more if stored in a tightly covered container in the refrigerator.*

- *Be sure the surface of the Roasted Garlic Paste is covered thoroughly with a layer of olive oil during storage, as this creates an airtight seal that helps preserve the paste.*

- *A toaster oven works very well for roasting the garlic, so you don't have to heat your entire large oven for just this one small item.*

▶ **YIELD: ABOUT 3 ONE-TABLESPOON SERVINGS**
Protein: 3 g / Saturated Fat: 2 g /
Polyunsaturated Fat: 1 g /
Monounsaturated Fat: 10 g /
Dietary Fiber: 1 g / Calories: 186

1. Preheat the oven to 375°F. Line a small baking sheet with foil and pour a little olive oil (about ½ teaspoon) onto each spot where you plan to place a bulb of garlic.

2. Slice off just the very tips of the garlic bulbs (a fraction of a fraction of an inch), and discard. Otherwise, leave the bulbs intact and unpeeled.

3. Place the bulbs cut-side-up on the oiled spots. Drizzle the top of each bulb with ½ to 1 teaspoon additional oil, and place the baking sheet on the center rack of the oven.

4. Roast for 30 minutes, or until the bulbs feel soft when gently pressed. (Larger bulbs will take longer.) Remove the baking sheet from the oven and let it stand while the garlic cools.

5. When the bulbs are cool enough to handle, simply break each one into individual cloves, and squeeze out the roasted garlic pulp into a small bowl. This process will be a little sticky. It will also be highly aromatic.

6. Mash the pulp with a fork, adding about 1 tablespoon additional olive oil as you mix. Transfer to a clean, dry container with a tight-fitting lid, smooth out the top of the paste, and drizzle with enough additional oil to make a film that covers the entire surface. Cover and refrigerate until use.

Guacamole

Authentic guacamole is very simple to prepare—it's just pure, ripe avocados with touches of seasoning added. Although best known as a dip for chips, guacamole is tremendously versatile, providing a substantial, colorful accompaniment to many savory dishes, especially those featuring eggs, beans, tomatoes, or cornmeal.

1 tablespoon fresh lemon or lime juice

1 large firm, ripe avocado (about 5 to 6 ounces)

Pinch of salt

Pinch of ground cumin

1 tablespoon minced red onion

2 tablespoons minced fresh tomato or tomato-based salsa

Cayenne

- *This keeps for only a day or so, tightly covered and refrigerated, but is best eaten right after it's made.*

▶ YIELD: 4 SERVINGS (ABOUT 2 TABLESPOONS PER SERVING)

Protein: 1 g / Saturated Fat: 1 g / Polyunsaturated Fat: 1 g / Monounsaturated Fat: 4 g / Dietary Fiber: 3 g / Calories: 76

1. Place the lemon or lime juice in a medium-small bowl. Cut the avocado in half, remove the pit, and scoop the flesh into the bowl.

2. Use a fork to slowly mash the avocado into the juice, adding the salt and cumin as you go.

3. When the avocado reaches your desired consistency (and that could well include a few lumps), stir in the onion and tomato or salsa. Add cayenne to taste. Serve right away—or soon.

Avocado "Butter"

Avocado lovers are always relieved and excited to learn that their favorite green comfort food not only is permitted on this diet, but is actually encouraged! This is a great way to make it into a simple sandwich spread or a dip for whole-grain crackers or vegetables. Just be sure the avocado you use is perfectly ripe, so it will mash effortlessly into a creamy, smooth consistency.

1 teaspoon fresh lime juice

1 small (3-ounce) avocado (or half a large one)

Salt

- *If you are using only half a larger avocado for this, you can preserve the other half by leaving in the pit, and drizzling the open surface with lemon juice. Wrap it tightly in plastic wrap and store out of direct light— either at room temperature (if your kitchen is not too hot) or in the refrigerator. Use this other half on a salad within a day or so—or just make a double batch of Avocado "Butter" to begin with!*

- *Store in a tightly covered container in the refrigerator. It will keep up to 2 days.*

▶ **YIELD: 2 SERVINGS (ABOUT 1½ TABLESPOONS PER SERVING)**
Protein: 1 g / Saturated Fat: 1 g / Polyunsaturated Fat: 1 g / Monounsaturated Fat: 4 g / Dietary Fiber: 3 g / Calories: 73

1. Pour the lime juice onto a plate.
2. Scoop out the avocado, directly into the lime juice.
3. Add a generous pinch of salt.
4. Mash with a fork until smooth.

Yogurt Cheese

With no fancy equipment whatsoever, you can become an artisan cheesemaker. Just drain a good deal of the liquid from any kind of yogurt, and the thickened result will be a soft and tasty homemade cheese. Simple and impressive! There are two ways to go about this low-tech process. The first approach uses a strainer, some cheesecloth, a bowl, and a bag of beans. The second method (for the many of you who don't happen to keep a supply of cheesecloth around on any kind of regular basis) calls for nothing more elaborate than drip coffee equipment, namely, a cone and a paper filter. Really and truly. The only disadvantage to this scheme is that you can't make a large amount at one time, because your "dripping space" is smaller. Yogurt Cheese will keep for 3 to 4 days if wrapped tightly and stored in the refrigerator.

Method One

2 cups plain nonfat yogurt

▶ YIELD: ABOUT 1 CUP (4 SNACK-SIZE SERVINGS)

Protein: 5 g / Saturated Fat: 0 g / Polyunsaturated Fat: 0 g / Monounsaturated Fat: 0 g / Dietary Fiber: 0 g / Calories: 50

1. Line a large strainer with a triple thickness of cheesecloth (cut a piece 10 inches long), and place it over a medium-size bowl.
2. Set the yogurt in the strainer, and fold the cheesecloth around it, wrapping it tightly, then place a weight on top. (A bag of dried beans works very well.)
3. Let stand for up to 24 hours, either at room temperature, or in the refrigerator, if your kitchen is very warm. About half the liquid will drain out. Tightly wrap the resulting cheese in plastic wrap, and refrigerate until use.

Method Two

1 cup plain nonfat yogurt

▶ YIELD: ABOUT ½ CUP (2 SNACK-SIZE SERVINGS)

Protein: 5 g / Saturated Fat: 0 g / Polyunsaturated Fat: 0 g / Monounsaturated Fat: 0 g / Dietary Fiber: 0 g / Calories: 50

1. Place a paper filter in a large-size (No. 6) drip coffee cone, and place the cone on a large mug, small bowl, liquid measuring cup, or any vessel over which it fits securely.
2. Add the yogurt, then just leave it alone. No weighting is required, as the whey (yogurt liquid) will drip out on its own.
3. Let stand for up to 24 hours, either at room temperature, or in the refrigerator, if your kitchen is very warm. About half the liquid will drain out. Tightly wrap the resulting cheese in plastic wrap, and refrigerate until use.

Tangy Black-Bean Dip

Add this very tasty concoction to your growing list of "dump and blend" recipes that come out tasting as though they were fussed over for hours!

¼ cup tomato juice

One 15-ounce can black beans, rinsed and drained (or 1¾ cups cooked black beans)

2 tablespoons fresh lime juice

½ to 1 teaspoon minced fresh garlic (start with less; see how you like it)

¾ teaspoon ground cumin

¼ teaspoon salt (or more to taste)

¼ teaspoon red pepper flakes (or more to taste)

Optional toppings:

Hot sauce

Salsa

Minced parsley and/or cilantro

- *Cooking tip: Roll the lime on the countertop, pressing it down, before you squeeze it for juice. This will maximize juice extraction!*

▶ **YIELD: ABOUT 2 CUPS (8 QUARTER-CUP SERVINGS)**
Protein: 3 g / Saturated Fat: 0 g /
Polyunsaturated Fat: 0 g /
Monounsaturated Fat: 0 g /
Dietary Fiber: 3 g / Calories: 53

1. Place all the ingredients except the optional toppings in a blender or food processor, and puree to a thick paste.
2. Taste to adjust garlic, then transfer to a container with a tight-fitting lid (or put it in a decorative bowl and cover tightly with plastic wrap). Refrigerate until serving time. Serve cold, with or without toppings. Keeps up to a week, refrigerated.

Hummus

You can buy very good prepared hummus in almost any grocery store or deli these days, but it is fun (and cheaper) to make your own.

Two 15-ounce cans chickpeas, rinsed and drained (or 3½ cups cooked chickpeas)

6 tablespoons sesame tahini

6 tablespoons fresh lemon juice

1 teaspoon minced garlic (or more, to taste)

½ teaspoon salt (or more, to taste)

1 teaspoon ground cumin

Cayenne

Extra-virgin olive oil, for the top

1. Place all ingredients except the cayenne and olive oil in a blender or food processor and puree to a thick paste.
2. Add cayenne to taste, and correct garlic and salt to your liking. (Keep in mind that the garlic will get stronger as the hummus sits around.)
3. Transfer to a container with a tight-fitting lid, and smooth the top. Pour a little olive oil on top, and tilt until it coats the surface completely. Cover and refrigerate until use.

- *This keeps for about a week if stored in a tightly covered container in the refrigerator.*

▶ **YIELD: 3½ CUPS (14 QUARTER-CUP SERVINGS)**

Protein: 5 g / Saturated Fat: 1 g / Polyunsaturated Fat: 2 g / Monounsaturated Fat: 2 g / Dietary Fiber: 4 g / Calories: 122

Tahini Sauce

Serve this classic Middle Eastern sauce over cooked vegetables or any main-dish protein.

5 tablespoons fresh lemon juice

¾ cup sesame tahini

½ teaspoon minced or crushed garlic (or more, to taste)

3 or 4 sprigs fresh parsley

½ teaspoon salt (or more, to taste)

About 1 cup water

Cayenne

• *This keeps for weeks if stored in a tightly covered container in the refrigerator.*

▶ **YIELD: ABOUT 1½ CUPS (12 TWO-TABLESPOON SERVINGS)**

Protein: 3 g / Saturated Fat: 1 g / Polyunsaturated Fat: 4 g / Monounsaturated Fat: 3 g / Dietary Fiber: 1 g / Calories: 93

1. Combine the lemon juice, tahini, garlic, parsley, and salt in a food processor fitted with a steep blade or a blender, and whip until uniform.

2. Keep the machine running as you slowly drizzle in the water. When all the water is incorporated, check the consistency. If you'd like it thinner, drizzle in a little extra water.

3. Transfer the sauce to a bowl or container. Add cayenne to taste, and possibly add more salt or garlic, if you like. (Keep in mind that the garlic will get stronger as the Tahini Sauce sits around.) Serve at room temperature or cold.

Spiced Yogurt

Add a little Indian-style seasoning and a scattering (or even a stampede) of fresh vegetables to a bowlful of yogurt, and you have a raita—a general term, in Indian cooking, for yogurt sauces served as a cooling contrast to spicy curries. This is also a wonderful sauce for many other things (you get to choose).

1 teaspoon whole cumin seeds

2 cups plain nonfat yogurt

¼ teaspoon salt

⅛ teaspoon cayenne

Up to 1 cup minced cucumber (peeled and seeded)

Optional Additions (Amounts are flexible; the more, the merrier!):

Minced bell pepper

Minced red onion

Grated carrot

Diced ripe tomato

Minced or torn cilantro leaves

- *Make this as close to serving time as possible. It keeps for only a day, or maybe two, but not longer—or at least, it doesn't keep well longer—in a tightly covered container in the refrigerator.*

▶ **YIELD: AT LEAST 2½ CUPS (OR MORE, DEPENDING ON HOW MANY EXTRA VEGETABLES YOU ADD)**

Protein: 4 g / Saturated Fat: 0 g / Polyunsaturated Fat: 0 g / Monounsaturated Fat: 0 g / Dietary Fiber: < 1 g / Calories: 45

1. Lightly toast the cumin seeds in a toaster oven or a small skillet over medium heat. Watch carefully to avoid burning. When the seeds give off a strong, toasty aroma, remove the pan from the heat.

2. Place the yogurt in a medium-size bowl, and add the whole toasted cumin seeds, along with the salt, cayenne, and cucumber—and whatever optional additional vegetables you prefer, leaving out the tomato and cilantro until the last possible minute. Mix until thoroughly blended.

3. Serve cold, topped with a scattering of diced tomato and minced or torn cilantro leaves, if desired.

Balsamic Glaze

Balsamic vinegar is reduced to a thick, flavorful syrup when cooked down to about two thirds of its original volume. You can drizzle this amazing stuff over more foods than you'd ever imagine—everything from roasted vegetables and grain dishes to all forms of Protein-of-Choice. It's even great on pancakes, fruit, and frozen desserts. This might just be the most versatile one-ingredient sauce ever.

1 cup balsamic vinegar

- *You don't need to use an expensive brand of vinegar for this recipe. In fact, the ordinary, more moderately priced supermarket varieties work the best.*

- *Store Balsamic Glaze in a covered container in the refrigerator or at room temperature. Theoretically, it will keep forever, but undoubtedly you will use it up sooner than that. If it hardens, just zap it in a microwave for a few seconds and it will soften right up again.*

▶ YIELD: ⅓ CUP
(5 ONE-TABLESPOON SERVINGS) (EASILY MULTIPLIED)
Protein: < 1 g / Saturated Fat: 0 g / Polyunsaturated Fat: 0 g / Monounsaturated Fat: 0 g / Dietary Fiber: 0 g / Calories: 31

1. Place the vinegar in a small, nonaluminum saucepan (a shallow one, if possible) and heat to boiling. (You might want to open your kitchen windows to vent the fumes!)
2. Turn the heat way down, and simmer uncovered for about 30 minutes, or until the vinegar is reduced in volume by about two thirds.
3. Transfer to a bowl, cover tightly, and store indefinitely at room temperature.

Pomegranate-Lime Glaze

Pomegranate molasses is a delicious condiment available at Middle Eastern food shops—or in the imported-foods section of basic grocery stores. It keeps forever in your cupboard, and a little bit goes a long way. In this simple sauce (which also keeps forever, if refrigerated) pomegranate molasses is just mixed with some fresh lime juice for a stunning result. It's good on all vegetables, grains, tofu, chicken, meat—you name it.

¼ cup pomegranate molasses

1 tablespoon plus 1 teaspoon fresh lime juice

▶ **YIELD: ⅓ CUP (5 ONE-TABLESPOON SERVINGS)**
Protein: 0 g / Saturated Fat: 0 g / Polyunsaturated Fat: 0 g / Monounsaturated Fat: 0 g / Dietary Fiber: 0 g / Calories: 33

Combine the two ingredients in a small bowl, and mix with a spoon or a small whisk until smooth. Serve at room temperature, spooned over hot or room-temperature food.

Sesame-Mustard Glaze

You can spoon this tangy little condiment onto any Protein-of-Choice to give it a boost. It's also a really good sandwich spread. This keeps for weeks if stored in a tightly covered container in the refrigerator.

3 tablespoons Dijon mustard

1 tablespoon Chinese-style toasted sesame oil

3 tablespoons orange juice (freshly squeezed, if possible)

1 tablespoon light-colored honey

1 tablespoon extra-virgin olive oil

A touch of minced fresh cilantro (optional)

▶ **YIELD: ½ CUP (8 ONE-TABLESPOON SERVINGS)**
Protein: < 1 g / Saturated Fat: < 1 g / Polyunsaturated Fat: 1 g / Monounsaturated Fat: 2 g / Dietary Fiber: 0 g / Calories: 48

Combine everything in a small bowl, and mix with a spoon or a small whisk until well blended. Cover and refrigerate until serving time.

Dark Sweet and Sour Sauce

This sauce is delicious on vegetables, and also on all protein choices, grains, and noodles. It's a good basic sauce to include in your cooking repertoire.

1½ teaspoons cornstarch

½ cup water

1 tablespoon low-sodium soy sauce

1 tablespoon plus 1 teaspoon cider vinegar

1 tablespoon plus 1 teaspoon light-colored honey

½ teaspoon Chinese-style toasted sesame oil

1 teaspoon grated fresh ginger

1 teaspoon minced or crushed garlic

- *This sauce keeps well for up to 2 weeks in a tightly covered container in the refrigerator, but will need to be stirred from the bottom and reheated gently before serving.*

▶ YIELD: ½ CUP
(2 SERVINGS)

Protein: 1 g / Saturated Fat: 0 g / Polyunsaturated Fat: < 1 g / Monounsaturated Fat: < 1 g / Dietary Fiber: 0 g / Calories: 70

1. Place the cornstarch in a small saucepan.
2. Drizzle in the water, whisking until the cornstarch dissolves.
3. Whisk in all the remaining ingredients, then place the pot on the stove over medium heat.
4. Heat to the boiling point, whisking constantly. Just before the sauce boils, turn the heat down to a simmer, and keep whisking for 2 to 3 minutes, or until slightly thickened and very smooth.
5. Serve hot or warm over vegetables, or other savory foods.

Amazing Gravy

With only two ingredients and in just 10 minutes you can make a perfect gravy. It's important that the broth itself be delicious, as this becomes the flavor of the gravy. So use your own best homemade, or go for one of those really good commercial brands that come unrefrigerated in 1-quart boxes. One excellent brand is Imagine, which makes a very good vegetable broth and also a No-Chicken Broth, both of them organic. (See page 171 for more details about broth.)

2 cups delicious broth

2 tablespoons unbleached all-purpose flour

Salt (optional)

Freshly ground black pepper (optional)

• *Keep this in a tightly covered jar in the refrigerator, and use as needed over the period of a week. You can also freeze it.*

▶ **YIELD: 4 SERVINGS**

Protein: 1 g / Saturated Fat: 0 g /
Polyunsaturated Fat: 0 g /
Monounsaturated Fat: 0 g /
Dietary Fiber: 1 g / Calories: 22

1. In a medium-size saucepan, heat the broth until it is hot, but not boiling.
2. Place the flour in a small bowl, and ladle in enough broth to dissolve the flour (approximately ¾ cup). Use a small whisk to beat this mixture until smooth, then pour it back into the hot broth. Whisk the broth as you pour.
3. Cook over medium heat, stirring frequently, for 5 to 8 minutes, or until lightly thickened. Add salt and pepper to taste, if desired.

Amazing Mushroom Gravy

Please see the notes about broth on the opposite page.

¼ pound mushrooms

1 tablespoon canola oil

Pinch of dried thyme

¼ teaspoon salt (or more, to taste)

1 teaspoon minced or crushed garlic

2 cups delicious broth

2 tablespoons unbleached all-purpose flour

Freshly ground black pepper (optional)

- *Keep this in a tightly covered jar in the refrigerator and use as needed over a period of a week. You can also freeze it.*

▶ YIELD: 4 SERVINGS

Protein: 2 g / Saturated Fat: < 1 g / Polyunsaturated Fat: 1 g / Monounsaturated Fat: 2 g / Dietary Fiber: 1 g / Calories: 61

1. Clean the mushrooms and, if the stems are firm and tight, leave them on. If they are soft and beginning to separate, remove and discard them. Chop the mushrooms into very small pieces, or, if you prefer, you can cut them into thin slices.

2. Place a medium-size saucepan over medium heat for 30 seconds. Add the oil and swirl to coat the pan. Add the mushrooms, thyme, and salt, and sauté for about 8 to 10 minutes, or until the mushrooms are reduced in size and they have expressed some juices. Stir in the garlic.

3. Add the broth, and heat until it is hot, but not boiling.

4. Place the flour in a small bowl, and ladle in enough broth to dissolve the flour (approximately ¾ cup). Use a small whisk to beat this mixture until smooth, then pour it back into the hot broth. Whisk the broth as you pour.

5. Cook over medium heat, stirring frequently, for 5 to 8 minutes, or until lightly thickened. Add salt and pepper to taste, if desired.

Mollie's Vinaigrette

Here's your basic salad dressing, a beautiful workhorse that you can make in just seconds with only four ingredients. Please note that the fresher the garlic, the better this will taste.

½ teaspoon minced or crushed garlic

¼ teaspoon salt

3 tablespoons balsamic or sherry vinegar

½ cup plus 2 tablespoons extra-virgin olive oil

- *This keeps for months, if stored in a tightly covered container in the refrigerator.*

▶ YIELD: ABOUT ⅔ CUP (11 ONE-TABLESPOON SERVINGS)

Protein: 0 g / Saturated Fat: 2 g / Polyunsaturated Fat: 1 g / Monounsaturated Fat: 9 g / Dietary Fiber: 0 g / Calories: 111

1. Measure the garlic, salt, and vinegar into a small bowl or a jar with a tight-fitting lid.
2. Use a small whisk to stir until well blended.
3. Keep whisking as you drizzle in the oil in a steady stream. The mixture will thicken as the oil becomes incorporated.
4. Cover tightly, and refrigerate until use. Immediately before using, shake well or stir from the bottom.

Roasted Garlic Vinaigrette

Roasted Garlic Paste is needed for this recipe, so make it ahead of time—and keep making it! It's a terrific staple to have on hand, and it keeps for a month or longer in the refrigerator.

1 tablespoon Roasted Garlic Paste (page 185)

¼ teaspoon salt

3 tablespoons balsamic or sherry vinegar

½ cup plus 2 tablespoons extra-virgin olive oil

▶ YIELD: ⅔ CUP (11 ONE-TABLESPOON SERVINGS

Protein: 0 g / Saturated Fat: 2 g / Polyunsaturated Fat: 1 g / Monounsaturated Fat: 9 g / Dietary Fiber: 0 g / Calories: 117

1. Measure the Roasted Garlic Paste, salt, and vinegar into a small bowl or a jar with a tight-fitting lid. Use a small whisk to stir until well blended.
2. Keep whisking as you drizzle in the oil in a steady stream. The mixture will thicken as the oil becomes incorporated.
3. Cover tightly, and refrigerate until use. Immediately before using, shake well or stir from the bottom.

Buttermilk Ranch Dressing

A really good alternative to that ever-popular staple, this is the cleanest version around! It keeps for a week or more, if stored in a tightly covered container in the refrigerator.

½ cup low-fat buttermilk

2 to 3 tablespoons mayonnaise (any kind)

1 teaspoon cider vinegar

½ teaspoon onion powder (or to taste)

¼ teaspoon garlic powder (or to taste)

⅛ teaspoon salt (or to taste)

Freshly ground black pepper

1. Measure all ingredients except the black pepper into a small bowl or a jar with a tight-fitting lid.
2. Use a small whisk to mix until uniform.
3. Taste to adjust salt and grind in some black pepper to taste.
4. Cover tightly, and refrigerate until use. Immediately before using, shake well or stir from the bottom.

▶ YIELD: A GENEROUS ½ CUP (8 ONE-TABLESPOON SERVINGS)

Protein: 1 g / Saturated Fat: < 1 g / Polyunsaturated Fat: 1 g / Monounsaturated Fat: < 1 g / Dietary Fiber: 0 g / Calories: 25

Creamy Balsamic Dressing

Sometimes you just want some creaminess in your basic vinaigrette. This one tastes luxurious and rich, especially if you add the optional shallot (a wonderful flavor-cross between mild, sweet onion and garlic). Store it in a tightly covered container in the refrigerator, and it will keep for several weeks.

2 tablespoons balsamic vinegar

4 tablespoons low-fat buttermilk

2 tablespoons light-colored honey

⅛ teaspoon salt (or more, to taste)

1 to 2 teaspoons finely minced shallot (optional)

5 tablespoons extra-virgin olive oil

1. Measure the vinegar, buttermilk, honey, salt, and shallot into a small bowl or a jar with a tight-fitting lid.
2. Use a small whisk to mix until uniform.
3. Keep whisking as you drizzle in the oil in a steady stream. The mixture will thicken as the oil becomes incorporated. Adjust the salt to taste.
4. Cover tightly, and refrigerate until use. Immediately before using, shake well or stir from the bottom.

▶ YIELD: ABOUT ¾ CUP (12 ONE-TABLESPOON SERVINGS)

Protein: 0 g / Saturated Fat: 1 g / Polyunsaturated Fat: 1 g / Monounsaturated Fat: 4 g / Dietary Fiber: 0 g / Calories: 64

Honey-Mustard Dressing

In addition to its more conventional use on salads, this really good dressing doubles as a sparkling sauce on any Protein-of-Choice (pages 201–210). Delicious and different!

2 to 3 tablespoons balsamic or sherry vinegar

2 tablespoons Dijon mustard

½ teaspoon minced or crushed garlic

⅛ teaspoon salt

2 teaspoons light-colored honey

6 tablespoons extra-virgin olive oil

• *This dressing keeps for weeks—and even months—if stored in a tightly covered container in the refrigerator.*

▶ **YIELD: ABOUT ½ CUP (8 ONE-TABLESPOON SERVINGS)**

Protein: 0 g / Saturated Fat: 1 g / Polyunsaturated Fat: 1 g / Monounsaturated Fat: 8 g / Dietary Fiber: 0 g / Calories: 110

1. Measure 2 tablespoons of the vinegar into a small bowl or a jar with a tight-fitting lid.
2. Use a small whisk to stir constantly as you add the mustard, garlic, salt, and honey.
3. Keep whisking as you drizzle in the oil in a steady stream. The mixture will thicken as the oil becomes incorporated.
4. Taste to see if you might like it a little sharper, and if so, add the additional tablespoon of vinegar.
5. Cover tightly, and refrigerate until use. Immediately before using, shake well or stir from the bottom.

Avocado-Yogurt Dressing

The acid from the fruit juice preserves the avocado's lovely green color. Use this luxurious dressing for Avocado Waldorf (page 160) or on any sliced fruit or green leafy salad.

¼ cup orange juice (fresh-squeezed, if possible)

1 tablespoon fresh lemon juice

1 small (3-ounce) avocado—or half a larger one, perfectly ripe

½ cup plain nonfat yogurt

1 tablespoon light-colored honey (possibly a little more)

Pinch of salt

Up to ½ teaspoon grated lemon zest or orange zest (optional)

• *This dressing will keep for about 3 days in a tightly covered container in the refrigerator.*

1. Combine the orange juice and lemon juice in a medium-size shallow bowl.
2. Scoop out the avocado and add it to the juice. Mash with a fork until very smooth.
3. Use a small whisk to beat in the yogurt and honey.
4. Add salt to taste, and some citrus zest, if you like. Stir and transfer to a container with a tight-fitting lid. Chill until serving time.

▶ **YIELD: ¾ CUP**

Protein: 1 g / Saturated Fat: 1 g / Polyunsaturated Fat: < 1 g / Monounsaturated Fat: < 1 g / Dietary Fiber: 1 g / Calories: 25

DINNER ENTRÉES

Protein-of-Choice

In addition to having a refrigerator full of fresh fruits and vegetables, and a cupboard filled with whole grains, legumes, and nuts, it's a good idea to keep ready-to-use cooked protein on hand as well. Many of the dinners on the 21-Day Diet suggest a "Protein-of-Choice." This option allows you to "fill in the blank" with your favorite protein, which, of course, can vary from night to night—and from week to week—as well it should.

Here are basic methods for cooking seven protein staples that work really well as the centerpiece for many of the dinners on our plans. These simple approaches are designed to get you going, and to acquaint beginning cooks with some of the fundamentals. If your cooking repertoire already includes these items (or you have a good and easy source for buying them prepared) you can go ahead and use your own favorite cooked tofu, chicken, meat, etc. And if you want to keep it ultra-simple, you can always swap in one cup low-fat cottage cheese, two eggs (any style), or a small can of tuna. For additional flavor, and to keep it interesting, you can adorn or augment any plain protein with any of the sauces, gravies, and glazes on pages 193 through 197 in a "mix and match" manner.

A single serving should be approximately the size of the palm of your hand. The yields on these recipes will approximate that, and approximation is fine. If the portion sizes vary slightly, that's okay. A little extra pure protein will not bust your diet—and in fact, can help keep you satisfied.

Basic Chicken Breast

For many people, keeping cooked chicken breast on hand is key to making a weight-control plan really work. You can toss it into main-dish salads, stir-fried vegetables, sandwiches, broths—anything. And once you cook it, it will keep for up to 5 days, if tightly wrapped and refrigerated. It keeps even better (and sometimes longer) if "preserved" in a little oil-and-vinegar-style salad dressing and stored in a tightly covered container. If you are a chicken eater, we strongly recommend keeping a good supply of boneless breasts in the freezer, and defrosting and cooking them on a regular basis as your Protein-of-Choice.

Here are the basic methods for cooking both bone-in and boneless chicken breasts.

Boneless, Skinless Chicken Breast Cutlet

One 4-ounce boneless, skinless chicken breast (a half breast)

Olive oil spray or extra-virgin olive oil as needed

Salt

Garlic powder

Poultry seasoning, or dried thyme and/or sage (optional)

▶ YIELD: 1 SERVING
Protein: 26 g / Saturated Fat: 2 g /
Polyunsaturated Fat: 2 g /
Monounsaturated Fat: 10 g /
Dietary Fiber: 0 g / Calories: 246

1. Place a heavy-bottomed, nonstick sauté pan or frying pan over medium-high heat for about 3 minutes. Generously spray the hot pan with olive oil spray, or add 1 tablespoon olive oil, and swirl to coat the pan.

2. Pat the chicken dry with paper towels, and sprinkle it lightly on both sides with salt, garlic powder, and a little poultry seasoning.

3. Place the chicken in the hot, oil-coated pan, and cook for 3 to 4 minutes on each side (depending on thickness). To test for doneness, just cut it open in the center and make sure it no longer looks pearly and shiny on the inside.

4. Remove from the pan immediately to stop cooking. Serve at any temperature.

Roasted Chicken Breast (on the bone)

1 medium-size half breast (bone in, skin on)—about ¾ pound raw weight

Olive oil spray or extra-virgin olive oil as needed

Salt

Freshly ground black pepper

Garlic powder

Poultry seasoning, or dried thyme and/or sage (optional)

Paprika

▶ YIELD: 2 SERVINGS

Protein: 32 g / Saturated Fat: 1 g / Polyunsaturated Fat: 1 g / Monounsaturated Fat: 5 g / Dietary Fiber: 0 g / Calories: 211

1. Preheat the oven to 400°F. Lightly coat a small baking pan with olive oil spray or olive oil.

2. Pat the chicken dry with paper towels, and brush or sprinkle it lightly on all sides with salt, pepper, garlic powder, and a little poultry seasoning.

3. Arrange the chicken skin-side-up in the prepared pan, and dust the top with paprika. Place on the center rack of the oven, and roast for 25 to 30 minutes, or until golden brown. To test for doneness, insert a sharp knife along the bone at the thickest part, and gently lift to see that there is no pearly-looking flesh visible. (A neater, easier, and more accurate way to check is to insert an instant-read meat thermometer into the thickest section. It should register 160°F.)

4. After removing the chicken from the oven, you can "tent" a small piece of foil over it for about 5 minutes, to increase its juiciness.

Basic Tofu

Tofu comes in so many forms these days it is hard to standardize any conversation about it, let alone a recipe. That said, a rule of thumb about tofu is that the firmer it is, the more nutritious. The simple logic here is that when more water is out of the curd, more pure substance remains. The calorie count will therefore be greater in firm tofu than in soft, but so will the amount of protein. In other words, with firmer tofu, you are getting more *food*. If you prefer softer tofu, that's fine. Just eat about 50 percent more of it, to be sure you are getting enough nutrition.

Here are the three forms of tofu that work best as a Protein-of-Choice selection in the 21-Day Diet:

1. Baked Tofu — Ready to Eat!

This comes in shrink-wrapped packages in the refrigerated section of the supermarket or natural-foods grocery. Baked tofu is very firm, to the point of being downright chewy, and it is often quite nicely seasoned. This product is ready-to-eat, so you need do nothing to it—except perhaps slice it and heat it, if you want it hot. (It also tastes very good cold.) There are now many flavors of baked tofu, and most of them are delicious and savory. Buy several types and do some taste tests to discover your favorites. Usually the net weight of shrink-wrapped firm tofu is 8 ounces, and you can consider three-fourths of that (6 ounces) to be two servings of Protein-of-Choice. (You can use the extra 4 ounces on a salad or in miso soup, etc. The part you don't eat right away can be stored in a tightly covered container in the refrigerator—not in water, once it's cooked—for up to 5 days.)

Protein: 25 g / Saturated Fat: 0.5 g /
Polyunsaturated Fat: 1.5 g /
Monounsaturated Fat: 1.55 g /
Dietary Fiber: 1 g / Calories: 170

2. Nigari Tofu

Similar to baked tofu, this ultra-firm variety usually comes in little 8-ounce, shrink-wrapped "bricks." It is completely unseasoned, so it needs a little boost in your kitchen. Prepare the entire package at one time, and consider it to be one serving, plus a little extra. Six ounces, or three-fourths of it, make one Protein-of-Choice serving. As with Baked Tofu, you can use the extra on a salad or in miso soup, etc. Once again, the part you don't eat right away can be stored in a tightly covered container in the refrigerator (not in water, once it's cooked) for up to 5 days.

One 8-ounce block nigari tofu
Nonstick spray or canola oil
Salt
Garlic powder

▶ YIELD: ABOUT 1¼ SERVINGS

Protein: 15 g / Saturated Fat: 2 g /
Polyunsaturated Fat: 8 g /
Monounsaturated Fat: 8 g /
Dietary Fiber: 1 g / Calories: 240

1. Place a heavy-bottomed, nonstick sauté pan, griddle, or frying pan over medium-high heat for about 3 minutes. Generously spray the hot pan with nonstick spray, or add 1 tablespoon canola, and swirl or brush to coat the pan.

2. Cut the tofu into rectangles or triangles about 2 inches by 1½ inches and a little more than ¼-inch thick. Pat it dry with paper towels, and sprinkle lightly all over with salt and garlic powder.

3. Place the tofu on the hot, oil-coated surface, and cook for 5 to 8 minutes on each side, or until golden and slightly crisp. You can decide when it's done, as tofu is a precooked product anyway. Serve at any temperature.

3. Firm Tofu (the kind that comes in a tub of water)

Even though the label says "firm," this kind of tofu still contains quite a bit more water than does the nigari variety. So firm it up further, and then cook it exactly as described in the preceding nigari method. To firm up already-firm tofu, cut the block into quarters, and simmer it in gently boiling water for 10 minutes. Drain well, and follow the preceding recipe. A 1-pound piece of firm tofu will yield about 2 servings.

Protein: 16 g / Saturated Fat: 1 g /
Polyunsaturated Fat: 5 g /
Monounsaturated Fat: 5 g /
Dietary Fiber: 1 g / Calories: 204

Basic Cooked Fish

Many different types of fish cook similarly if they are of comparable size and shape, so this is pretty much a "one method fits all" primer. Actually, make that three methods. These are the most straightforward approaches for broiling, sautéing, and "oven-finishing" a 1-inch-thick fish steak or fillet. Each takes only 10 minutes or less.

One 6-ounce fresh fish fillet or steak (1 inch thick)

Olive oil spray or extra-virgin olive oil as needed

Salt

- *If you are cooking thinner, more delicate fish, you can use the same methods, but the cooking time will be reduced by up to half. When broiling thinner fillets, you might want to line the pan with a piece of oiled foil.*

▶ **YIELD: 1 SERVING**

Protein: 35 g / Saturated Fat: 2 g / Polyunsaturated Fat: 3 g / Monounsaturated Fat: 11 g / Dietary Fiber: 0 g / Calories: 306

To Broil:

1. Adjust the oven rack so that the surface of the fish will be about 4 inches from the heat. Preheat the broiler to 500°F. Place the broiler pan in the hot oven for about 5 minutes.

2. Spray the hot pan with olive oil spray or brush it liberally with olive oil. Pat the fish dry with paper towels, place it skin-side-down in the pan, and spray or brush its top surface with additional oil. Sprinkle lightly with salt.

3. Broil on the first side for 3 to 5 minutes, until it turns golden brown, and the flesh is just turning from translucent to opaque.

4. Turn the fish over, and broil for another 3 to 5 minutes on the second side. When done, the top surface should just begin to flake when nudged gently with a fork. It's okay if it seems a little rare, as the fish will continue to cook once removed from the broiler. Serve right away.

To Sauté:

1. Place a heavy-bottomed, nonstick sauté pan or frying pan over medium-high heat for about 3 minutes. Generously spray the hot pan with olive oil spray, or add 1 tablespoon olive oil, and swirl to coat the pan.

2. Pat the fish dry with paper towels, and place it skin-side-down in the hot, oil-coated pan. Spray or brush the top surface of the fish with additional oil, and sprinkle lightly with salt.

3. Sauté on the first side for 3 to 5 minutes, until it turns golden brown and the flesh is just turning from translucent to opaque.

4. Turn the fish over, and sauté for another 3 to 5 minutes on the second side. When done, the top surface should just begin to flake when nudged gently with a fork. It's okay if it seems a little rare, as the fish will continue to cook once removed from the heat. Serve right away.

To "Oven-Finish":

1. Preheat the oven to 400°F.

2. Follow the sauté method above, making sure the pan you use has an ovenproof handle.

3. After you turn over the fish, transfer the pan to the oven for 3 to 5 minutes, depending on how well cooked you like your fish. Do err on the side of underdone, as the fish will continue to cook once removed from the oven. Serve right away.

Basic Beef

The best way to prepare beef as your Protein-of-Choice is to broil it. And if you will be broiling meat on any kind of regular basis, it's a good idea to invest in an instant-read meat thermometer, to help you cook it until perfectly (and not too) done.

½ pound flank steak, London broil, or another very lean beef steak—1 inch thick

1 tablespoon extra-virgin olive oil

Salt

Garlic powder

- *After beef is cooked, it will keep best if left unsliced, so wrap the unused portion tightly in plastic wrap and then place it in a resealable plastic bag and refrigerate for 3 to 4 days.*

▶ **YIELD: 2 SERVINGS**

Protein: 31 g / Saturated Fat: 9 g / Polyunsaturated Fat: 1 g / Monounsaturated Fat: 13 g / Dietary Fiber: 0 g / Calories: 350

1. Adjust the oven rack so that the surface of the beef will be about 4 inches from the heat. Preheat the broiler to 500°F and preheat the broiler pan for about a minute, as well.

2. Trim and discard all visible excess fat from the steak, and pat the meat dry with paper towels.

3. Brush the surface of the meat all over with olive oil, and sprinkle lightly all over with salt and garlic powder. Place on the preheated broiler pan.

4. Broil for 4 minutes or until nicely browned on the first side, then turn over and broil for the same amount of time on the second side. The meat is done when an instant-read thermometer registers about 130° to 135°F. (Cooking past 140°F will toughen the meat.)

5. Transfer the meat to a carving board and let it rest, tented with foil, for about 5 minutes before slicing. Slice off just the amount you wish to eat, then wrap the rest in plastic wrap and place it in a resealable plastic bag and store in the refrigerator.

Basic Tempeh

Originally from Indonesia, tempeh is a firm, chewy, fermented "cake" made from partially cooked soybeans (sometimes with grain added) that have been inoculated with spores and then aged. It is a very versatile, high-protein food that can be used in a wide range of savory dishes. Look for tempeh in the refrigerator or freezer section of natural-food stores, shrink-wrapped in 8-ounce packages. If it's frozen, defrost before using.

Tempeh is a partially cooked product, and needs to be cooked further before it is edible. After years of experimenting, Mollie has found this browning treatment to be the very best way to go about it. When you brown tempeh in hot oil in an uncrowded pan, it becomes crunchy on the outside, and chewy on the inside, with a delightful nutty-toasty flavor.

1 tablespoon extra-virgin olive oil

8 ounces tempeh, cut into ½-inch dice

Nonstick spray (optional)

1 tablespoon balsamic vinegar

Freshly ground black pepper (optional)

- *You can make Basic Tempeh up to several days ahead of time. Store it in a tightly covered container in the refrigerator, and reheat it shortly before serving, in a hot pan lightly sprayed with nonstick spray, or in a microwave.*

▶ **YIELD: 2 SERVINGS**

Protein: 21 g / Saturated Fat: 3 g / Polyunsaturated Fat: 5 g / Monounsaturated Fat: 8 g / Dietary Fiber: 0 g / Calories: 284

1. Place a medium-size skillet or sauté pan over medium-high heat for about 2 minutes. Add the oil, wait another 10 seconds or so, then swirl to coat the pan.

2. When the cooking surface is hot enough to sizzle a bread crumb, add the tempeh and spread it into a single layer. Let it cook for a good 10 to 12 minutes, stirring occasionally, until it turns golden brown on all surfaces. If the tempeh appears to be sticking, push it to one side, lightly spray the pan with nonstick spray, then resume sautéing until all surfaces are golden.

3. Sprinkle in the vinegar, letting it hit the hot surface of the pan (it makes a great sizzling sound!), so it can reduce slightly on contact. Stir and cook over medium heat for another 5 minutes or so.

4. Serve hot, warm, or at room temperature, dusted with freshly ground black pepper to taste.

Basic Seitan

Seitan is wheat gluten, plain and simple. It doesn't sound very attractive, but it is actually a delightfully chewy high-protein food with a pleasantly neutral flavor. When sliced and lightly sautéed, it takes on the textural properties of chicken or beef. In fact, there are brands of seitan that even bill it as a chicken or meat analogue, and rightly so. You can purchase seitan in shrink-wrapped 8-ounce packages—or packed in broth—in the refrigerator section of natural-food groceries (usually with or near the tofu).

1 tablespoon extra-virgin olive oil

8 ounces seitan, cut in ¼-inch slices

A generous splash of vegetable broth (optional)

- *Seitan keeps for months unopened, and once you prepare this basic recipe, it will keep for another week if tightly covered and stored in the refrigerator.*

- *The vegetable broth in this recipe is optional, but adds a nice touch of moisture and flavor. You can use a good commercial brand (such as Imagine) or, if the seitan you purchased came packed in its own broth, it's fine to use that. Keep in mind, though, that seitan-package broth is usually on the salty side.*

1. Place a medium-size skillet or sauté pan over medium heat for about 2 minutes. Add the oil, wait another 10 seconds or so, then swirl to coat the pan.
2. When the cooking surface is hot enough to sizzle a bread crumb, add the seitan and spread it into a single layer. Cook for 5 to 8 minutes, shaking the pan occasionally, until it becomes crisp on both sides.
3. Splash in a little vegetable broth, if desired, and let it cook for about a minute over medium heat, so it will partially evaporate.
4. Serve at any temperature.

▶ **YIELD: 2 SERVINGS**

Protein: 41 g / Saturated Fat: 1 g / Polyunsaturated Fat: 1 g / Monounsaturated Fat: 5 g / Dietary Fiber: 1 g / Calories: 246

Easy Three-Bean Chili

This makes a lot! Refrigerate or freeze any extra in a tightly covered container. (Freezing it in individual serving-size containers can be very convenient for future spontaneous dinners.) It reheats well.

2 tablespoons extra-virgin olive oil

1½ cups small-diced onion

1 cup diced bell peppers (a mix of red, yellow, and green is nice)

¼ teaspoon salt (or to taste)

2 tablespoons chili powder

1 tablespoon minced or crushed garlic

2 teaspoons ground cumin

1 teaspoon dried oregano

1 teaspoon dried basil

Big pinch of cayenne pepper

One 28-ounce can crushed tomatoes packed in tomato puree

One 15-ounce can diced tomatoes

1 cup vegetable broth

One 15-ounce can black beans, drained and rinsed

One 15-ounce can garbanzo beans, drained and rinsed

One 15-ounce can red kidney beans, drained and rinsed

Freshly ground black pepper

▶ YIELD: 10 SERVINGS
Protein: 10 g / Saturated Fat: 1 g /
Polyunsaturated Fat: 1 g /
Monounsaturated Fat: 2 g /
Dietary Fiber: 10 g / Calories: 211

1. Place a large saucepan or soup pot over medium-high heat and wait 2 minutes. Add the oil and wait about 30 seconds, then add the onion, peppers, and salt. Cook, stirring often, for 5 to 8 minutes, or until the onions are translucent and both the onions and peppers are beginning to soften.

2. Add the chili powder, garlic, cumin, oregano, basil, and cayenne; sauté until fragrant, about 1 minute.

3. Stir in the crushed tomatoes, diced tomatoes, and vegetable broth, and bring to a boil.

4. Add all the beans, and bring to a boil again. Reduce the heat, partially cover the pot, and let the chili simmer gently for 20 minutes—or as long as 1 hour. (If simmering longer, give it a stir every 10 minutes or so to see if it needs some additional stock.)

5. Grind in some black pepper, and taste to adjust the salt. Serve hot.

Mushroom-Barley Burgers

Here is a delicious departure from other vegetable burgers. Cook the barley well ahead of time. One cup of raw barley should yield 3 cups cooked. (See page 55.) You can use freshly cooked, still-warm barley in the mixture, but make sure it isn't steaming hot. These are tender burgers that you need to handle carefully, so they won't fall apart. However, if they do crumble a bit, you can push them back together as they cook—or just enjoy the crumbles!

1 tablespoon extra-virgin olive oil

2 cups minced onion

½ pound mushrooms, minced

1 teaspoon salt (or to taste)

2 tablespoons minced or crushed garlic

2 tablespoons balsamic vinegar

3 cups cooked pearl barley

½ cup minced, toasted walnuts

4 large eggs, beaten

1 packed cup grated part-skim mozzarella cheese

Freshly ground black pepper

Nonstick spray for the pan

- *Refrigerating the mixture for a few hours will help make these a little sturdier, but this step is purely optional.*

- *Uncooked burgers will keep for up to 2 days if tightly wrapped and refrigerated. Cooked burgers will keep for up to a week, tightly wrapped, in the refrigerator— and for months in the freezer.*

1. Place a large nonstick sauté pan or skillet over medium-high heat for 2 minutes. Add the oil, wait another 30 seconds or so, then add the onion. Cook, stirring occasionally, until translucent and beginning to soften, about 5 minutes.

2. Add the mushrooms and the salt. Cook, stirring often, for about 10 minutes, or until the liquid that the mushrooms exude has evaporated and they are beginning to take on some color.

3. Add the garlic and cook until fragrant, about 1 minute longer.

4. Remove from the heat and stir in the vinegar.

5. In a large bowl, combine the onion and mushroom mixture with the cooked barley and nuts. Add the eggs and mozzarella and stir well to combine.

6. Season with a few grinds of black pepper, then let the mixture sit for about 10 minutes at room temperature—or overnight in a tightly covered container in the refrigerator.

   At this point you can either fry the burgers on the stove-top, or bake them in the oven.

To fry the burgers on the stove-top:

1. Heat a large nonstick sauté pan or skillet over medium heat. When the pan is hot, generously spray with nonstick spray.

2. Using a ½-cup dry measuring cup, make 2 or 3 mounds of mixture, placing them directly into the hot pan. Leave yourself a

bit of room around each to make flipping them easier. Carefully flatten each mound to form 4-inch patties.

3. Cook without moving until nicely browned on the bottom, about 5 minutes. Carefully insert a thin-bladed spatula (it should be at least as wide as the patties, so it can support them) under the patties, first loosening them completely and then flipping them over, quickly but carefully.

4. Cook until nicely browned on the second side, about 5 minutes. Serve hot or warm.

To cook the burgers in the oven:

1. Preheat the oven to 400°F and place a non-stick baking sheet in the heating oven for a few minutes. Generously spray the heated baking sheet with nonstick spray.

2. Using a ½-cup dry measuring cup, make 2 or 3 mounds of mixture, placing them directly onto the hot baking sheet. Leave yourself a bit of room around each to make flipping them easier. Carefully flatten each mound to form 4-inch patties.

3. Place on the center rack of the oven and bake undisturbed for 10 minutes. Carefully insert a thin-bladed spatula (it should be at least as big as the patties, so it can support them) under the patties, first loosening them completely and then flipping them over, quickly but carefully.

4. Bake until nicely browned on the second side, about 10 minutes. Serve hot or warm.

▶ YIELD: 8 BURGERS (1 PER SERVING)

Protein: 11 g / Saturated Fat: 3 g /
Polyunsaturated Fat: 4 g /
Monounsaturated Fat: 4 g /
Dietary Fiber: 3 g / Calories: 233

Madras Vegetable Curry

A medley of colorful vegetables in a highly seasoned sauce provides a great backdrop for any plain Protein-of-Choice (pages 201–210) and also works well on its own. You can use any curry powder you like, keeping in mind that they are all different. You might want to make this dish a number of times with different curry powders, to discover your favorite (a fun project!).

1 tablespoon canola oil or peanut oil

2 cups chopped onion

2 tablespoons curry powder

½ teaspoon salt (or to taste)

2 medium sweet potatoes (about 6 ounces each), peeled and cut into bite-size pieces

2 medium carrots, sliced or diced

1 small cauliflower, cut or broken into ½-inch florets

1 cup vegetable broth or water (possibly more)

One 15-ounce can diced tomatoes

One 5- or 6-ounce package fresh baby spinach leaves

1 cup nonfat yogurt

- *You can make this curry with vegetable broth or water. If you use broth, choose a high-quality store-bought brand.*

- *After you add the yogurt, the sauce might curdle a little, but just keep mixing, and it will be fine (and taste great).*

- *Leftovers will keep for up to a week in a tightly covered container in the refrigerator.*

▶ YIELD: 5 SERVINGS

Protein: 7 g / Saturated Fat: < 1 g / Polyunsaturated Fat: 1 g / Monounsaturated Fat: 2 g / Dietary Fiber: 7 g / Calories: 172

1. Place a large saucepan or soup pot over medium-high heat and wait 2 minutes. Add the oil and wait about 30 seconds, then add the onion, curry powder, and salt. Cook, stirring often, for 5 to 8 minutes, or until the onion is translucent and beginning to soften.

2. Stir in the sweet potatoes, carrots, and cauliflower, making sure they get completely coated with the curried onions, and sauté for another 3 minutes or so.

3. Stir in the vegetable broth and tomatoes, and bring to a boil. Lower the heat to a simmer, partially cover the pot, and cook gently for another 8 to 10 minutes, or until all the vegetables are tender.

4. Add the spinach, and give it a stir. The spinach will wilt within seconds.

5. Stir in the yogurt and remove from the heat. Serve hot.

Broiled Eggplant Parmesan

Unlike the traditional version, which has the eggplant battered and fried, and then baked in a casserole, this quick, clean version is made under the broiler in just a few steps. It's fun to prepare, and really delicious. Be sure to use a good commercial tomato sauce (or your own favorite homemade) and high-quality Parmesan cheese, freshly grated, if possible.

Extra-virgin olive oil as needed

2 small Japanese, Chinese, or Baby Italian eggplants (about 6 ounces each)

Salt

Freshly ground black pepper

6 tablespoons good-quality tomato sauce

6 tablespoons part-skim ricotta cheese

6 tablespoons shredded part-skim mozzarella cheese

1 tablespoon grated Parmesan cheese

3 tablespoons minced fresh basil (optional)

- *This will keep for only about 2 days if covered tightly and refrigerated, and is best eaten right after it's made.*

▶ **YIELD: 2 SERVINGS**

Protein: 12 g / Saturated Fat: 5 g / Polyunsaturated Fat: 1 g / Monounsaturated Fat: 7 g / Dietary Fiber: 1 g / Calories: 228

1. Preheat the broiler to 500°F and move the oven rack to the highest position. Lightly brush a baking sheet with olive oil.

2. Cut the eggplants in half lengthwise, and place each half cut-side-up on the prepared baking sheet.

3. Lightly brush the cut surface of each eggplant half with olive oil, then broil until the top is golden and fork-tender (about 5 to 6 minutes). Turn the eggplant halves over, and broil on the second side until very soft, another 5 to 6 minutes or so.

4. Remove the eggplants from the broiler and lower the oven rack to the second highest position.

5. Turn the eggplants cut-side-up, and sprinkle lightly with salt and pepper. Spread each half of the eggplant with 1½ tablespoons tomato sauce, then spoon 1½ tablespoons ricotta over each half in an even layer. Sprinkle each half with 1½ tablespoons mozzarella and ½ tablespoon Parmesan.

6. Return to the broiler and cook until the cheeses are melted and have formed a lovely golden brown crust, about 5 to 7 minutes. Serve immediately, topped with a sprinkling of minced fresh basil.

Buckwheat Noodles
with Cashews and Greens

Slender, dark, flavorful buckwheat noodles (also known as soba) are available in Japanese food shops and in natural-food groceries. They are chewy and complex, and combine beautifully with cooked greens and toasted cashews for a very satisfying, quickly prepared one-dish microwave meal.

1 tablespoon light-colored honey

1 tablespoon cider vinegar

2 teaspoons low-sodium soy sauce

4 ounces uncooked Japanese-style buckwheat noodles

One 10-ounce package baby spinach leaves (or two 5-ounce packages) or 10 ounces small-leaf mixed braising greens, coarsely chopped

2 tablespoons Chinese-style toasted sesame oil

1 teaspoon minced or crushed garlic

Salt

½ cup chopped cashews, lightly toasted

Red pepper flakes

- *This dish will keep for at least 5 days if stored in a tightly covered container in the refrigerator.*

▶ YIELD: 3 SERVINGS

Protein: 12 g / Saturated Fat: 4 g / Polyunsaturated Fat: 6 g / Monounsaturated Fat: 10 g / Dietary Fiber: 4 g / Calories: 402

1. Place the honey in a small bowl. Add the vinegar and soy sauce, and stir until the honey dissolves. Set aside.

2. Bring a large pot of water to a boil. Add the noodles and cook until tender (about 4 minutes).

3. Meanwhile, place the prepared greens in a medium-large microwave-safe bowl.

4. When the noodles are done, drain them and immediately add them to the greens in the bowl. Add the sesame oil and garlic, and mix with a fork or tongs, bringing up the greens from the bottom so that they wilt from the contact with the hot noodles.

5. Place the bowl in a microwave, and cook on high for one minute to further wilt the greens.

6. Remove from the microwave, and add the honey–soy sauce–vinegar mixture. Stir with the fork or tongs as you add salt to taste.

7. Sprinkle the top with cashews and red pepper flakes, if desired, and serve hot, warm, or at room temperature.

Baked Stuffed Peppers Filled
with Bulgur–Pine Nut Pilaf

Get a little fancy on a weeknight with this elegant dish—and lift your spirits in the process. It's not a lot of work, especially if you make the pilaf well ahead of time.

Extra-virgin olive oil as needed

4 medium-size (6-ounce) bell peppers

1 recipe Bulgur–Pine Nut Pilaf (page 240)

- *Use warm-colored (red, yellow, and/or orange) bell peppers, if you can. They are much sweeter—and lovelier, visually—than green ones.*

- *Once baked, these will keep for up to a week if wrapped tightly and refrigerated. They reheat really well in a microwave or regular oven.*

▶ **YIELD: 4 SERVINGS**

Protein: 2 g / Saturated Fat: 1 g / Polyunsaturated Fat: < 1 g / Monounsaturated Fat: 4 g / Dietary Fiber: 4 g / Calories: 106

1. Preheat the oven to 375°F. Lightly oil a baking sheet.

2. Use a sharp paring knife to cut the stem from each pepper, reserving the stems. Reach inside the peppers with the knife or a spoon to scrape out the pith and seeds. Do your best to leave the peppers intact in the process.

3. Spoon in ½ cup pilaf per pepper, patiently packing it down as you go. Place the stems back on top as a plug for the filling (or, if you want to get poetic, as a hat for the pepper).

4. Brush the outside surface of each pepper with a little additional olive oil, and place them standing upright, if possible, on the prepared baking sheet.

5. Bake for 35 minutes on the center rack of the oven. Serve hot or warm.

Green Beans in Crunchy Peanut Coating
with Protein-of-Choice

"Fun" is not usually the adjective we use to describe a dinner entrée. Here's an exception.

The fresher and firmer the green beans, the better this will taste. There are two cooking processes involved—toasting and seasoning the peanuts, followed by a dramatic green-bean stir-fry. You can save on labor by using the same pan for both, although it will seem a bit large for the relatively small volume of peanuts.

¾ cup peanuts (unsalted)

2 tablespoons peanut oil or canola oil

2 tablespoons minced fresh ginger

½ teaspoon grated lemon zest

1 pound fresh green beans, trimmed and cut into 1½-inch pieces

½ teaspoon salt (or to taste)

2 servings Protein-of-Choice (pages 201–210), cut into strips or bite-size pieces

1 tablespoon minced or crushed garlic

1 tablespoon fresh lemon juice

Red pepper flakes

• *Have ready 2 palm-size servings of any Protein-of-Choice, cut into strips or bite-size pieces.*

▶ YIELD: 3 SERVINGS

Protein: 29 g / Saturated Fat: 3 g / Polyunsaturated Fat: 6 g / Monounsaturated Fat: 9 g / Dietary Fiber: 9 g / Calories: 345

1. Place the peanuts in a blender, and grind briefly in a few bursts, until they form a coarse meal. Set aside.

2. Place a large, heavy-bottomed, nonstick sauté pan or large frying pan over medium heat for about 2 minutes. When it is hot, add about 2 teaspoons of the oil. Wait another 10 seconds or so, then swirl to coat the middle section of the pan. (It won't be enough oil to reach all the way to the edges.)

3. Add the ginger, and sauté for a few minutes, then add the crushed peanuts and the lemon zest. Cook over medium-low heat for about 10 minutes, stirring often, until the peanuts are lightly toasted. Transfer to a dish, and return the pan to the stove over medium heat. (You don't need to clean the pan at this point.)

4. After the pan has been sitting over medium heat for 3 minutes, add the rest of the oil, wait another 10 seconds, then swirl to coat the pan.

5. Turn the heat to high, and add the green beans and salt. (The pan should sizzle when the green beans hit.) Stir-fry over high heat for about 5 minutes, or until "tender-crisp," shaking the pan and using tongs to keep the green beans moving as they cook.

6. Stir in the Protein-of-Choice along with the garlic. Lower the heat to medium, and cook for another 2 to 3 minutes, or until everything is heated through.
7. Toss in the lemon juice and the peanut mixture, and stir until well combined. Sprinkle lightly with red pepper flakes, and serve right away.

Vegetable-Almond Fried Rice

If you set up everything ahead of time, with all your ingredients by the stove and ready, this stir-fry will go really quickly. Just heat the wok or skillet and begin! Cook the rice as much as several days ahead of time. You will need 3 cups of cooked brown rice, which is approximately 1 cup raw, cooked in 1¾ cups water (details are on page 54). This dish will keep for several days if stored in a tightly covered container in the refrigerator.

1 teaspoon plus 2 tablespoons peanut oil or canola oil

2 large eggs, beaten

1 large bunch broccoli, chopped into ½-inch pieces

1 large onion, chopped (about 2 cups chopped)

2 large carrots, sliced on the diagonal or diced

½ teaspoon salt

½ pound firm tofu, diced, or 1 cooked chicken half breast, diced (pages 202–203)

1 small (6-inch) zucchini or yellow summer squash, diced

1 to 2 tablespoons minced garlic

3 cups cooked long-grain brown rice (page 54)

1 cup peas (frozen/defrosted)

4 medium scallions, minced (whites and greens)

Low-sodium soy sauce

1 cup coarsely chopped or slivered almonds, lightly toasted

Condiments:

Extra soy sauce

Chinese-style toasted sesame oil

Red pepper flakes and/or chili oil

▶ YIELD: 6 SERVINGS

Protein: 19 g / Saturated Fat: 2 g / Polyunsaturated Fat: 5 g / Monounsaturated Fat: 10 g / Dietary Fiber: 10 g / Calories: 400

1. Place a large wok or skillet over medium heat and wait about 30 seconds. Add 1 teaspoon oil and swirl to coat the pan. Add the beaten eggs, and slowly tip the pan in all directions, allowing the eggs to spread into a thin layer. Keep tilting until the eggs have reached their limit and are cooked through. Use a spatula to transfer the cooked eggs to a plate, then cut the eggs into small pieces or strips with a dinner knife.

2. Wipe the wok or skillet clean with a paper towel and return it to high heat. Wait another 30 seconds, then add 2 tablespoons oil and swirl to coat the pan. Add the broccoli, onion, carrots, and salt, and cook for 5 minutes, stirring constantly.

3. Add the tofu or chicken, zucchini or summer squash, and more or less garlic, depending on your taste. Turn the heat down to medium, and stir-fry another 3 minutes or so, until the vegetables are all "tender-crisp."

4. Fork in the rice a little at a time, as you keep the mixture moving over medium heat. When all the rice is in, dump in the peas and scallions, and shake in about 20 good shakes of soy sauce, as you stir and cook for just a minute longer. Stir in the almonds.

5. Serve hot, and pass shakers of condiments.

Thai-Inspired Green Curry

Really good, authentic Thai ingredients are widely available in many American grocery stores these days, thanks to a growing interest in ethnic foods. The best and most readily accessible brand is Thai Kitchen, so look for their products in the "international" section where you buy your food. This dish is intensely seasoned! (The Thai Kitchen green curry paste is not for the faint palate!) However, it gets toned down and balanced by the soothing coconut milk. Use this curry as a sauce for any Protein-of-Choice (pages 201–210) or eat it on its own as you would a soup—or with a little brown basmati rice.

1 cup light coconut milk

1 cup vegetable broth or chicken stock

1 teaspoon green curry paste

One 3-inch piece of lemongrass, cut in two, then split lengthwise, or 1½ teaspoons grated lemon zest

2 tablespoons Thai fish sauce (*nam pla*) (optional)

1 small yellow summer squash (about 4 ounces), cut into ½-inch-thick half-rounds

1 cup (about 4 ounces) zucchini, cut into ½-inch-thick half-rounds

1 cup small broccoli florets

2 tablespoons minced fresh cilantro (optional)

1. In a medium saucepan, combine the coconut milk, broth or stock, and green curry paste. Whisk to combine.
2. Add the lemongrass or lemon zest. Bring to a boil over high heat, then reduce the heat and simmer, covered, for 15 minutes.
3. Remove and discard the lemongrass stalk, if using. Stir in the fish sauce. Add the squash, zucchini, and broccoli, and bring to a boil. Reduce the heat and simmer, uncovered, until the vegetables are just tender. Serve hot, sprinkled with cilantro if desired.

• *This dish will keep for only about a day or two, and is best eaten fresh. If you need to store it, refrigerate it in a tightly covered container and reheat it gently.*

▶ **YIELD: 3 SERVINGS**
Protein: 4 g / Saturated Fat: 1 g /
Polyunsaturated Fat: < 1 g /
Monounsaturated Fat: < 1 g /
Dietary Fiber: 3 g / Calories: 67

Thai-Inspired Red Curry

As with Thai-Inspired Green Curry, this makes a great sauce for any Protein-of-Choice (pages 201–210). You can eat it on its own as you would a soup—or with a little brown basmati rice.

1 cup light coconut milk

½ cup vegetable broth or chicken stock

1 teaspoon red curry paste

1 teaspoon minced fresh ginger

2 tablespoons fish sauce (*nam pla*) (optional)

2 teaspoons brown sugar (optional)

1 cup canned diced tomatoes, drained

1 cup (about 3 ounces) Japanese or Chinese eggplant, cut into ½-inch thick half-rounds

1 cup (about 4 ounces) green beans, cut into 2-inch lengths

2 tablespoons minced fresh basil (Thai basil, if available)

1. In a medium saucepan, whisk together the coconut milk, broth or stock, red curry paste, and ginger. Bring to a boil over high heat, reduce the heat, and simmer, covered, for 15 minutes.
2. Stir in the fish sauce and brown sugar, if using. Add the diced tomatoes and eggplant. Bring to a boil, then reduce the heat and simmer, uncovered, until the eggplant is tender.
3. Add the green beans and simmer until tender. Serve hot, topped with minced fresh basil.

- *Thai-Inspired Red Curry will keep for only about a day or two, and is best eaten fresh. If you need to store it, refrigerate it in a tightly covered container and reheat it gently.*

▶ YIELD: 3 SERVINGS

Protein: 2 g / Saturated Fat: 2 g / Polyunsaturated Fat: < 1 g / Monounsaturated Fat: < 1 g / Dietary Fiber: 4 g / Calories: 84

VEGETABLE SIDE DISHES

Slow-Roasted Roma (Plum) Tomatoes

In this recipe, you are gently and gradually rendering the tomatoes in your oven, shrinking them over a period of more than 2 hours into chewy sweetness, as their juices evaporate and their natural sugars caramelize. Dressed lightly with olive oil, they are as nutritious as they are sensuous.

1 to 2 tablespoons extra-virgin olive oil

2 pounds medium-size Roma tomatoes (3 to 4 ounces each) (If you use smaller ones, you can just halve them.)

- *The long oven time notwithstanding, Slow-Roasted Roma Tomatoes actually require very little work. So plan to make them on an evening or afternoon when you are at home anyway, doing other things.*

- *These will keep for about 5 days in a tightly covered container in the refrigerator.*

▶ **YIELD: 6 TO 8 SMALL SERVINGS OF A FEW SLICES EACH**

Protein: 1 g / Saturated Fat: < 1 g / Polyunsaturated Fat: < 1 g / Monounsaturated Fat: 3 g / Dietary Fiber: 2 g / Calories: 57

1. Preheat the oven to 275°F. Line a baking sheet with foil and brush with 1 tablespoon of the olive oil.

2. Core the tomatoes and halve them lengthwise, then cut them in half again to make long quarters.

3. Arrange the tomato slices skin-side-down on the prepared baking sheet. It's okay if they are touching.

4. Place the baking sheet on the center rack of the oven. After an hour or so, the tomatoes will have stuck slightly to the foil. Loosen them gently with a small spatula and/or by shaking the baking sheet.

5. Repeat this process of moving around and jostling every 10 minutes or so for the second hour. At some point, turn the tomatoes over, using tongs.

6. You get to decide when they're done—but let this be at least 2½ hours after they've been in the oven.

7. When the tomatoes are done to your liking, remove them from the oven and let them cool to room temperature directly on the foil. Transfer to a storage container with a tight-fitting lid, and drizzle the tops with a little extra olive oil. Refrigerate and use as desired, cold or at room temperature.

Apple-Glazed Acorn Squash Rings

Simple and sweet, with a broiled top, these golden circles will literally round out your dinner plate.

Nonstick spray for the pan

One medium-size acorn squash (about 1⅓ pounds)—skin on, seeds removed, cut into ½-inch rings

3 tablespoons apple juice or defrosted apple juice concentrate (or more)

- *Be careful slicing the squash. Use a very sharp paring knife, inserting the point first, and using a gentle sawing motion.*

- *The easiest way to remove the seeds is to cut loose the strand around them with scissors, and then scrape them away with a spoon.*

▶ **YIELD: 3 SERVINGS (ABOUT 3 PIECES PER SERVING)**
Protein: 1 g / Saturated Fat: 0 g / Polyunsaturated Fat: 0 g / Monounsaturated Fat: 0 g / Dietary Fiber: 2 g / Calories: 69

1. Preheat the oven to 375°F.
2. Line a baking sheet with foil, and spray it lightly with nonstick spray.
3. Arrange the squash rings on the prepared baking sheet, and place on the center rack of the oven.
4. After 15 minutes (or when the squash is fork-tender), remove the baking sheet from the oven and drizzle or brush the squash with apple juice or apple juice concentrate.
5. Heat the broiler to 500°F and move the oven rack to the highest position. Place the baking sheet under the broiler for just a minute or two, until the squash tops begin to brown. (Watch carefully—they can burn quickly.) Remove from the oven, and if desired, glaze with a touch more apple juice or concentrate. Serve hot, warm, or at room temperature.

A Sparkling Sweet Potato

An exciting discovery: All you need to add to a cooked sweet potato, for an utterly divine result, is a healthy drizzle of fresh lime juice. That's all! No butter, no salt. And absolutely no marshmallows. The title of this recipe is singular; it actually allows you to make a single serving at a time. This presupposes you'll be making this often and/or making an extra few to share with others, who will be envious of your diet when they get a taste.

1 medium-size sweet potato (about 6 ounces)

1 to 2 tablespoons fresh lime juice (or to taste)

- *This will keep for up to a week in a tightly covered container in the refrigerator.*

▶ **YIELD: 1 SERVING**
Protein: 2 g / Saturated Fat: 0 g / Polyunsaturated Fat: 0 g / Monounsaturated Fat: 0 g / Dietary Fiber: 3 g / Calories: 95

1. Place the sweet potato in a microwave, and cook for 3 minutes on high. Turn it over, and repeat for another 3 minutes. Insert a fork into the center of the sweet potato to test for doneness. It should go in easily. If it doesn't, cook for another minute or two. (You can also roast the sweet potato in a 375°F oven until fork-tender.)

2. Remove the sweet potato from the microwave (or oven), and let it cool until comfortable to handle. Peel off the skin by hand (it should come off easily).

3. Transfer the peeled sweet potato to a small bowl, and mash by hand with a fork. As you mash, add 1 tablespoon of the lime juice.

4. Keep mashing until the lime juice is distributed, then give it a taste. Add more lime juice as needed.

5. Serve warm or at room temperature—or reheat it in the microwave and serve it hot.

Roasted Butternut Squash

In some grocery stores, you can find peeled and cut butternut squash in the produce department, shrink-wrapped in plastic. If this appeals to you, go ahead and take this shortcut. No one will know that you didn't peel and cut a fresh squash yourself.

1 tablespoon canola oil or saf-flower oil

1 pound butternut squash

Salt (optional)

- *Roasted Butternut Squash will keep for up to 5 days in a tightly covered container in the refrigerator, and will respond beautifully to all sorts of sauces, glazes, and salad dressings.*

▶ **YIELD: 3 SERVINGS (A GENEROUS ½ CUP PER SERVING)**

Protein: 2 g / Saturated Fat: < 1 g / Polyunsaturated Fat: 1 g / Monounsaturated Fat: 3 g / Dietary Fiber: 4 g / Calories: 97

1. Preheat the oven to 425°F. Line a baking sheet with parchment paper or foil, and brush or spread it with some of the oil.
2. Peel the squash, then cut it in half. Scrape out and discard the few seeds, and chop the squash into 1-inch cubes.
3. Distribute the squash cubes on the prepared baking sheet, and brush the exposed sides with a little extra oil.
4. Place the baking sheet on the center rack of the oven, and roast for 10 minutes. Shake the baking sheet and/or use tongs to redistribute the squash so it can roast evenly all over.
5. Roast for another 10 minutes, then remove from the oven, and let the squash cool for about 10 minutes on the baking sheet. You can salt it lightly during this time, if you wish. Serve hot, warm, or at room temperature.

Roasted Asparagus

This is the ultimate way to prepare asparagus! You can roast asparagus of any thickness. Just keep your eye on it, and take it out of the oven before it is completely tender, as it will keep cooking from its own heat for another few minutes or so, and you don't want asparagus to get too soft.

1 tablespoon extra-virgin olive oil (possibly more)

1 pound asparagus, ends trimmed or snapped off

Salt (optional)

• *Roasted Asparagus will keep for up to 5 days if tightly covered and refrigerated, and will respond beautifully to all sorts of sauces, glazes, and salad dressings.*

▶ **YIELD: 3 SERVINGS**
Protein: 3 g / Saturated Fat: 1 g /
Polyunsaturated Fat: < 1 g /
Monounsaturated Fat: < 1 mg /
Dietary Fiber: 3 g / Calories: 80

1. Preheat the oven to 425°F. Line a baking sheet with parchment paper or foil, and brush or spread it with some of the oil.

2. Distribute the asparagus on the prepared baking sheet, and roll them around so they will be completely coated with oil.

3. Place the baking sheet on the center rack of the oven, and roast for 3 minutes. Shake the baking sheet and/or use tongs to redistribute the asparagus, so it can roast evenly all over.

4. After another couple of minutes in the oven, begin checking for doneness. Remove from the oven as soon as the asparagus is "this side of tender." You can salt it lightly, if you wish.

5. Serve hot, warm, or at room temperature. Roasted asparagus also tastes good cold.

Roasted Brussels Sprouts or Cauliflower

If you think you dislike either of these vegetables, think again. Or don't think at all, just go get some and roast them, and by then, everything will likely have changed. Crisp on the outside, and soft and savory on the inside, Roasted Brussels Sprouts and Roasted Cauliflower are both downright revelatory!

1 tablespoon extra-virgin olive oil (possibly more)

¾ pound brussels sprouts or cauliflower florets (1-inch pieces)

Salt (optional)

- This recipe can also be used for broccoli or for carrots. (Cut broccoli into medium spears and carrots into 1-inch chunks.)

- Whichever vegetable you roast, it will keep for up to 5 days in a tightly covered container in the refrigerator, and will respond beautifully to all sorts of sauces, glazes, and salad dressings.

▶ YIELD: 3 SERVINGS (A GENEROUS ½ CUP PER SERVING)
Protein: 3 g / Saturated Fat: 1 g / Polyunsaturated Fat: 1 g / Monounsaturated Fat: 3 g / Dietary Fiber: 3 g / Calories: 84

1. Preheat the oven to 425°F. Line a baking sheet with parchment paper or foil, and brush or spread it with some of the oil.

2. If roasting brussels sprouts, cut them in half. If they are very large, cut them into quarters. Place them cut-side-down on the prepared baking sheet, making sure all the cut surfaces touch some of the oil. With cauliflower, just dump the pieces on the baking sheet and shake them into a single layer.

3. Place the baking sheet on the center rack of the oven, and roast for 10 minutes. At this point, shake the baking sheet and/or use tongs to redistribute the vegetables so that more surfaces can come into contact with the hot, oiled baking sheet. This crisps everything up quite nicely!

4. Roast for another 5 minutes, or until a taste test tells you the vegetables are done to your liking. (They will cook a little further from their own heat after they come out of the oven.)

5. Remove from the oven, and let the vegetables cool for about 10 minutes on the baking sheet. You can salt them lightly during this time, if you wish.

6. Serve hot, warm, or at room temperature. Roasted vegetables also taste good cold.

One-Minute Spinach

It's very easy to just pop open a package of prewashed baby spinach and dump it into a pot (or a bowl, if you are using the microwave). One minute later, you will have a delicious and nutritious vegetable side dish. It will be even more delicious if you use flavorful vegetable broth, such as Imagine brand, and dress the final product with some tasty oil.

2 tablespoons vegetable broth or water

One 10-ounce package baby spinach leaves (or two 5-ounce packages)

Optional:

Salt

A drizzle of extra-virgin olive oil or a toasted nut oil or seed oil

A touch of minced or crushed garlic

- *One-Minute Spinach will keep for up to 5 days in a tightly covered container in the refrigerator.*

- *You can also make this with a 10-ounce package of frozen, defrosted spinach. Squeeze out some of the water after the frozen spinach has thawed.*

▶ YIELD: 2 SERVINGS (1 GENEROUS ½ CUP PER SERVING)

Protein: 3 g / Saturated Fat: 0 g / Polyunsaturated Fat: 0 g / Monounsaturated Fat: 0 g / Dietary Fiber: 7 g / Calories: 61

1. Place the broth or water and spinach in a medium-size microwave-safe bowl (if using a microwave) or pot (if using the stove). Cover the bowl with a plate—or the pot with a lid.

2. Microwave the bowl on high for 1 minute—or cook the spinach in the pot over medium-high heat for 1 minute.

3. Remove from the heat, and dress with a little salt, some oil, and/or a touch of garlic, if desired. Serve hot, warm, or at room temperature.

Spinach with Pine Nuts and Raisins

Once you get the hang of One-Minute Spinach (previous page), you need only go a short step further to create this impressive side dish. This will be even more delicious if you use flavorful vegetable broth, such as Imagine brand.

2 tablespoons vegetable broth or water

One 10-ounce package baby spinach leaves (or two 5-ounce packages)

Pinch of salt

2 teaspoons extra-virgin olive oil

½ teaspoon minced or crushed garlic

2 tablespoons pine nuts, lightly toasted

2 tablespoons raisins

Freshly ground black pepper

- This dish will keep for up to 5 days in a tightly covered container in the refrigerator.

- You can also make this with a 10-ounce package of frozen, defrosted spinach. Squeeze out some of the water after the frozen spinach has thawed.

▶ YIELD: 2 SERVINGS (1 GENER-OUS ½ CUP PER SERVING)

Protein: 5 g / Saturated Fat: 1 g / Polyunsaturated Fat: 3 g / Monounsaturated Fat: 5 g / Dietary Fiber: 8 g / Calories: 187

1. Place the broth or water and spinach in a medium-size microwave-safe bowl (if using a microwave) or pot (if using the stove). Cover the bowl with a plate—or the pot with a lid.

2. Microwave the bowl on high for 1 minute—or cook the spinach in the pot over medium-high heat for 1 minute.

3. Remove from the heat, and stir in the salt, olive oil, and/or garlic. Serve hot, warm, or at room temperature, topped with pine nuts, raisins, and a grind or two of fresh black pepper.

Braised Greens with Walnuts and Sour Cherries

Tart fruit is a welcome surprise in savory dishes—especially this one, where the nicely pungent accent from the toasted walnuts rounds it all out. The result is surprisingly balanced and smooth.

To braise is to cook in liquid. It's a process that's similar to steaming, only the liquid is in contact with the food it is cooking, so it goes a little faster. Also, if the liquid is flavorful, that adds to the dish. For that reason, we strongly recommend using the vegetable broth option. The oil comes at the end, as a seasoning. Use a good, fruity, extra-virgin olive oil or an aromatic nut or seed oil (such as walnut oil or roasted pumpkinseed oil), which makes this dish absolutely delicious.

3 tablespoons vegetable broth or water (possibly more, as needed)

1 pound assorted fresh leafy greens, stemmed if necessary, and coarsely chopped

Pinch of salt

1 tablespoon extra-virgin olive oil or a nut oil or seed oil

¼ cup dried sour cherries, cut into small pieces if large

¼ cup minced walnuts, lightly toasted

- *A mixture of collards, mustard greens, and kale is particularly good, but you can also make this with spinach, escarole, beet greens, dandelion greens—just about any dark leaf.*

- *You can also use a "braising mix" sold in bulk in many produce departments, and also increasingly available packaged.*

- *The amount of greens called for might seem enormous, but don't forget they will cook down dramatically.*

1. Heat the broth or water in a medium-large skillet with a tight-fitting lid.

2. Add the greens and sprinkle them very lightly with salt. Cover the pan and cook over medium heat for about 5 minutes, or until the greens wilt. (Check the level of broth or water after about 2 minutes, to be sure there's enough liquid to prevent sticking or burning.)

3. Transfer to a serving dish, and toss with the oil and cherries. Serve hot or warm, topped with the walnuts.

▶ YIELD: 3 SERVINGS (ABOUT ¾ CUP PER SERVING)
Protein: 6 g / Saturated Fat: 1 g /
Polyunsaturated Fat: 4 g /
Monounsaturated Fat: 5 g /
Dietary Fiber: 4 g / Calories: 174

Italian-Style Pan-Sautéed Broccoli

This double process is a wonderful way to cook broccoli. First you blanch large pieces in boiling water, after which you can store the broccoli for up to 5 days in the refrigerator. (Added benefit: The broccoli lasts longer after this cooking process, and takes up less refrigerator space than when raw.) Then, just before serving, you give it a delicious warm-up in gently heated garlic-infused olive oil, for a perfect finish.

1 pound broccoli

2 to 3 tablespoons extra-virgin olive oil

1 teaspoon minced or crushed garlic

Salt

Freshly ground black pepper

Red pepper flakes (optional)

- *You can also follow this process for cooking green leafy vegetables, such as kale, collard greens, spinach, or escarole. Blanch them (with stems removed, but otherwise uncut) for only 30 seconds and skip the cold water rinse. Squeeze out all the moisture, and pack them into tight little green rolls. When it comes time to serve them, just slice the packed rolls with a sharp knife, separate the cut leaves with your fingers, and give them the hot olive oil bath for about 5 minutes. Your guests will think you are brilliant!*

▶ **YIELD: 4 SERVINGS**
Protein: 3 g / Saturated Fat: 1 g / Polyunsaturated Fat: 1 g / Monounsaturated Fat: 6 g / Dietary Fiber: 3 g / Calories: 108

1. Bring a large pot of water to boil. In the meantime, trim and discard the tough stem end of the broccoli, and slice the rest lengthwise, into about 6 hefty spears.

2. When the water boils, lower the heat to a simmer, and plunge in the broccoli for 2 minutes if you like your vegetables tender-crisp, or for 3 minutes if you like them tender-tender.

3. Drain in a colander, and then rinse the broccoli under cold running water to cool it down. Drain thoroughly, then dry the broccoli first by shaking it emphatically, and then patting it with paper towels. Transfer to a resealable plastic bag, seal it, and store until use. When you want to finish the broccoli and serve it, take it out of the refrigerator and let it come to room temperature.

4. About 15 minutes before serving time, place a large skillet over medium-low heat and add the olive oil. While you are waiting for it to heat, cut the broccoli into smaller pieces (whatever size and shape you prefer).

5. When the oil has become warm (after about 3 minutes), add the garlic and the broccoli, and heat it in the oil, turning it with tongs every few minutes. Continue with this for 5 to 8 minutes (possibly even a little longer) until the broccoli is heated through, cooked to your liking, and delightfully coated with the garlic and oil.

6. Add salt and pepper to taste, plus a sprinkling of red pepper flakes if you like, and serve hot or warm.

Spaghetti Squash

For a mild and very satisfying high-volume dish, spaghetti squash is a terrific choice. Spaghetti squash looks like a plain, large, yellowish-green oval with a hard, woody stem. Once cooked, the flesh falls apart into strands (hence the name), with a light and crunchy texture, a subtle, slightly sweet taste, and an ethereal light-golden color.

Nonstick spray for the baking sheet

One 3-pound spaghetti squash

2 tablespoons extra-virgin olive oil

1 small slice butter (about 1 teaspoon) (optional)

1½ cups minced onion

½ teaspoon dried sage

¼ teaspoon salt (or to taste)

Up to 1 tablespoon minced or crushed garlic (optional)

Freshly ground black pepper

- *You can prepare and bake the squash up to several days ahead of time. Store it in a tightly covered container (or in a resealable plastic bag) in the refrigerator until use.*

- *The finished dish will keep, tightly covered and refrigerated, for about 5 days.*

▶ **YIELD: ABOUT 8 SERVINGS (½ CUP PER SERVING BUT FEEL FREE TO EAT AS MUCH AS YOU'D LIKE!)**
Protein: 1 g / Saturated Fat: < 1 g / Polyunsaturated Fat: < 1 g / Monounsaturated Fat: 3 g / Dietary Fiber: 2 g / Calories: 82

1. Preheat the oven to 350°F. Line a baking sheet with parchment paper or foil, and spray lightly with nonstick spray.

2. Cut the squash in half lengthwise, and scrape out the seeds. (The easiest way to remove the seeds is to cut loose the strand around them with scissors, and then scrape them away with a spoon.)

3. Bake the halves facedown on a lightly oiled baking sheet for about 30 minutes, or until the skin can be pierced fairly easily with a fork. Remove the baking sheet from the oven, and turn the squash over, leaving it on the baking sheet until it cools enough so that it is comfortable to handle. Then scoop out the insides, discarding the skin, and combing through the flesh with a fork to separate the strands. Set the squash aside.

4. Place a large skillet or sauté pan over medium heat and wait for about 1 minute. Add the olive oil, and swirl to coat the pan. If desired, add the butter to the olive oil.

5. Add the onion and sage to the hot pan, and cook, stirring frequently, for 5 to 8 minutes—or until the onion is becoming golden. Stir in the garlic, if using, and then add the squash and salt. Use a fork or tongs to mix the squash into the onion.

6. When the squash is warmed through and everything is well combined, it's time to serve. This dish tastes best hot or warm.

Five-Minute Flash-Cooked Green Beans

Once the beans are trimmed, all you need is a large hot pan, and the rest is one big sizzling action!

2 tablespoons canola or safflower oil

1 pound whole green beans, trimmed

Pinch of salt

1 tablespoon minced or crushed garlic

Red pepper flakes

- *These will keep for up to a week in a tightly covered container (or a resealable plastic bag) in the refrigerator.*

▶ **YIELD: 6 SERVINGS**
Protein: 1 g / Saturated Fat: < 1 g /
Polyunsaturated Fat: 1 g /
Monounsaturated Fat: 3 g /
Dietary Fiber: 3 g / Calories: 64

1. Place a large wok or sauté pan over medium heat for about 1½ minutes.
2. Add the oil and swirl to coat the pan. The oil should be hot enough to sizzle a bread crumb on contact.
3. Turn the heat to high, and wait 20 seconds or so, then add the green beans, and a pinch of salt.
4. Cook over high heat, shaking the pan and/or using tongs to turn and move the beans so they cook quickly and evenly.
5. After 3 minutes, take a taste test and see if the beans are done to your liking. They should be relatively crunchy, but you get to decide. If you like them cooked a little more, keep going until they're your kind of tender.
6. Sprinkle in the garlic and some red pepper flakes, and cook for just a minute longer. Serve hot, warm, or at room temperature.

Broiled Eggplant, Bell Peppers, Onions, and Portobellos

The trick to this dish—other than possessing an adept sense of timing and a nice, large platter—is to have a batch of vinaigrette dressing at the ready, so you can soak the freshly cooked vegetables in intense flavor as soon as they come off the heat. (Unlike meats, vegetables respond best to marination after, not before, they are cooked.) A double batch of Mollie's Vinaigrette (page 198) will provide more than enough, and you can make this well ahead of time.

Nonstick spray for the pan

1-pound globe eggplants, cut into half-inch slices (no need to peel)

1 medium-large red onion, cut into sixths lengthwise (no need to peel this, either)

1 cup Mollie's Vinaigrette (page 198)

2 medium red or orange bell peppers, seeded and cut into thick strips

2 medium (4-inch diameter) portobello mushrooms— wiped clean, stemmed, and quartered

- *Once prepared, this dish will keep for a week or longer, if covered tightly with plastic wrap and kept in the refrigerator.*

- *This dish tastes good at any temperature, but is best at room temperarure. So if you make it the night before, remember to take it out in time to warm up a bit before serving.*

▶ **YIELD: 5 SERVINGS**
Protein: 2 g / Saturated Fat: 1 g /
Polyunsaturated Fat: < 1 g /
Monounsaturated Fat: 3 g /
Dietary Fiber: 1 g / Calories: 83

1. Preheat the broiler to 500°F and move the oven rack to the highest position. Line a baking sheet with foil, and spray generously with nonstick spray.

2. Arrange the slices of eggplant and wedges of onion in a single layer on the baking sheet, and broil on each side for 3 to 5 minutes, or until everything is fork-tender and the eggplant is nicely browned.

3. Meanwhile, pour about ½ cup Mollie's Vinaigrette onto a medium-size platter with a rim.

4. When they're done to your liking, transfer the eggplant and onions directly onto the puddle of vinaigrette on the platter, then spoon a little additional vinaigrette on top.

5. Place the peppers and portobellos on the same baking sheet (you might want to use fresh foil and/or another application of nonstick spray) and broil them in the same way. They might take a little longer than the eggplant and onions, but you get to decide when they're done.

6. Transfer the broiled peppers and mushrooms to the same platter, arranging them artfully, and dress them lightly with a few additional tablespoons of vinaigrette.

7. Serve at room temperature.

Broiled Baby Zucchini Boats
with Parmesan Crust

Small zucchini are tender and moist, and really fun to eat in large pieces (halves, in this case) that are anointed in the broiler with a crunchy cheese topping. This is a good, quick, last-minute vegetable dish that you can whip up on a weekday after work.

1 tablespoon extra-virgin olive oil

2 teaspoons minced garlic

4 small zucchini and/or summer squash (slender ones, about 6 inches long), halved lengthwise

Salt

Freshly ground black pepper

Grated Parmesan cheese

▶ YIELD: 4 TO 6 SERVINGS

Protein: 3 g / Saturated Fat: 1 g / Polyunsaturated Fat: < 1 g / Monounsaturated Fat: 2 g / Dietary Fiber: 1 g / Calories: 45

1. Preheat the broiler to 500°F and move the oven rack to the highest position.

2. Heat the olive oil in a large cast-iron skillet or a frying pan with an ovenproof handle. Add the garlic, and sauté over medium-low heat for only about 30 seconds, so it cooks but does not brown. (Browning garlic makes it bitter.)

3. Place the zucchini halves facedown in the pan and sprinkle lightly with salt and pepper.

4. Turn up the heat to medium-high, and sauté for about 5 minutes, or until the zucchini are just slightly tender when poked gently with a fork.

5. Turn over the zucchini, and sprinkle with Parmesan. (Don't worry if the Parmesan spills into the pan. It will melt into additional delicious crust.) Cook for just a minute or two more, then transfer the skillet to the broiler.

6. Broil for about 3 to 5 minutes, or until the cheese is melted and golden brown. Serve hot, and be sure to scrape up the spilled Parmesan from the bottom of the pan.

Zucchini and Sweet Onions
in Butter-Spiked Olive Oil

A very quick stove-top dish, this is a good example of how you can "spike" olive oil with butter. Both flavors shine through, and the result tastes deceptively rich.

1 tablespoon extra-virgin
   olive oil

1 small slice butter (about
   1 teaspoon)

1 cup chopped onion

Four 7-inch zucchini (about
   1 pound)

¼ teaspoon salt (possibly
   more)

1 teaspoon minced garlic

Black pepper

▶ YIELD: 5 SERVINGS

Protein: 3 g / Saturated Fat: 1 g /
Polyunsaturated Fat: < 1 g /
Monounsaturated Fat: 2 g /
Dietary Fiber: 2 g / Calories: 65

1. Place a medium-large heavy skillet over medium heat. After about a minute, add the olive oil and swirl to coat the pan. Add the butter, and let it melt into the oil, then swirl to coat again.

2. Keeping the heat at medium, add the onion and give the pan a shake to distribute it into the hot buttered oil.

3. While the onion cooks, cut the zucchini into ½-inch slices. If you like, you can cut the rounds into half-circles.

4. After the onion has cooked for about 5 minutes, add the cut zucchini and the salt. Keep cooking and stirring for about 2 minutes, then add half the garlic.

5. Cover the pan, and let cook, stirring a few times, for 5 minutes longer—or until tender to your taste. Remove the cover and stir in the remaining garlic, then taste to adjust salt. Serve hot or warm, topped with some black pepper.

GRAIN DISHES

Whole-Wheat Couscous
with Pistachios and Orange Zest

Couscous is a tiny pasta, so it isn't really a whole grain, even though it is generally thought of—and treated—as one. But regardless of its categorization, the whole-wheat version of couscous is high in protein and fiber, so it measures up well. And like its cousin, bulgur, whole-wheat couscous needs only to soak in hot or boiling water for about 30 minutes before it's ready to eat. So it's a true convenience food that should go on your menu often.

½ cup whole-wheat couscous

½ cup boiling water

2 tablespoons finely minced chives or scallion

½ teaspoon grated orange zest

Pinch of salt

3 tablespoons chopped pistachio nuts, lightly toasted

1. Place the couscous in a medium-small bowl.
2. Pour in the water and cover the bowl with a plate. Let stand 30 minutes
3. Stir in the chives or scallion and orange zest, and add a little salt to taste. Serve warm or at room temperature, topped with pistachio nuts.

- This dish will keep for up to a week if tightly covered and refrigerated.

▶ YIELD: 2 SERVINGS
(¾ CUP PER SERVING)
Protein: 6 g / Saturated Fat: 1 g /
Polyunsaturated Fat: 2 g /
Monounsaturated Fat: 3 g /
Dietary Fiber: 5 g / Calories: 175

Bulgur with Olive Oil and Lemon

Bulgur is precooked cracked wheat that requires no further cooking beyond a good soak in boiling water. Use a very small amount of water, so the result will be fluffy and slightly chewy—and never mushy. Also, with less water, the natural nutty flavor of the grain comes through more strongly.

½ cup bulgur

½ cup boiling water

1 tablespoon extra-virgin
   olive oil

1 tablespoon fresh lemon juice

Pinch of salt

Finely minced fresh parsley
   (optional)

1. Place the bulgur in a medium-small bowl.
2. Pour in the water and cover the bowl with a plate. Let stand 30 minutes
3. Stir in the olive oil and lemon juice, and add a little salt to taste.
4. Stir in the parsley and serve warm or at room temperature.

- *You can prepare this the day before and reheat in a microwave—or you can make it after work and eat it the same day.*

- *It keeps for up to a week if tightly covered and refrigerated.*

▶ **YIELD: 2 SERVINGS
(¾ CUP PER SERVING)**

Protein: 4 g / Saturated Fat: 1 g /
Polyunsaturated Fat: 1 g /
Monounsaturated Fat: 5 g /
Dietary Fiber: 6 g / Calories: 181

Bulgur–Pine Nut Pilaf

Sautéing the uncooked bulgur and pine nuts in oil before adding the water gives this dish a deeper, toastier flavor.

2 tablespoons extra-virgin olive oil

½ cup bulgur

¼ cup pine nuts

½ cup boiling water

1 tablespoon freshly squeezed lemon juice

Pinch of salt

1 teaspoon minced fresh dill

1 to 2 tablespoons finely minced chives or scallion

1 tablespoon currants (optional)

- *This keeps for up to a week if stored in a tightly covered container in the refrigerator.*

▶ **YIELD: 2 SERVINGS (¾ CUP PER SERVING)**

Protein: 4 g / Saturated Fat: 1 g / Polyunsaturated Fat: 1 g / Monounsaturated Fat: 5 g / Dietary Fiber: 7 g / Calories: 183

1. Heat 1 tablespoon of the oil in a medium-small skillet with a tight-fitting lid.
2. Add the uncooked bulgur and the pine nuts, and sauté over medium heat for about 5 minutes, or until it gives off a toasty smell. Keep stirring during this process to be sure the bulgur doesn't burn.
3. Pour in the water and place the lid on the pan. Let stand 30 minutes.
4. Stir in the second tablespoon of olive oil and the lemon juice, and add a little salt to taste.
5. Stir in the remaining ingredients, and serve warm or at room temperature.

Millet and Quinoa
with Toasted Sunflower Seeds

Crunchy, nutty, toasty . . . and easy! It's always nice to have a good use for these humble, highly nutritious grains. The purpose of all that fluffing activity in steps 3 and 4 is to ensure that you end up with a bowlful of tender, separate grains, instead of mush. So get out that fork, and seriously fluff.

¾ cup millet
¼ cup quinoa
1½ cups water
Pinch of salt
¼ cup sunflower seeds,
   lightly toasted

Possible garnishes:

Wedges of lemon, lime, or
   orange
Minced fresh parsley
Tiny cherry tomatoes

- *Delicious though it is, this dish is somewhat monochromatic, so garnish it with something colorful, such as citrus wedges, grated carrots, minced parsley, or cherry tomatoes.*

- *This dish keeps for up to 4 days stored in a tightly covered container in the refrigerator.*

▶ YIELD: 4 SERVINGS (¾ CUP
PER SERVING)
Protein: 8 g / Saturated Fat: 1 g /
Polyunsaturated Fat: 4 g /
Monounsaturated Fat: 1 g /
Dietary Fiber: 5 g / Calories: 233

1. Place the millet and quinoa in a strainer, and rinse thoroughly under cold running water. Transfer the grains to a small saucepan, and add the water and a small pinch of salt.

2. Place the pan over medium heat and bring to a boil. Cover, and turn the heat down as far as it will go, then simmer, covered, for 15 minutes.

3. Stir the millet and quinoa from the bottom of the pot with a fork, and keep fluffing the grains for a minute or two, then cover again, and continue to cook for about 5 minutes longer, or until the grains are perfectly tender.

4. Transfer to a bowl, and fluff from the bottom with a fork to let steam escape. Let stand uncovered for about 15 minutes, repeating the fluffing procedure every few minutes or so.

5. Stir in the toasted sunflower seeds, and serve warm or at room temperature with garnishes as desired.

Kasha Varnishkes

Buckwheat combined with pasta and seasoned simply with onion—this is the kind of food that, according to Mollie's mother, keeps body and soul together. It's also very quick and easy. If you have any left over, try it cold, as a snack. This keeps for up to 5 days in a tightly covered container in the refrigerator.

1 tablespoon extra-virgin olive oil

¾ cup minced onion

1 cup uncooked kasha or buckwheat groats

¼ teaspoon salt (or to taste)

1¼ cups boiling water

¾ cup uncooked small bow-tie pasta (whole grain, if possible)

2 to 3 scallions, minced

1 tablespoon fresh dill, minced

Freshly ground black pepper

- *"Kasha" simply refers to buckwheat that has been dry-roasted. Kasha and plain buckwheat groats can be used interchangeably.*

▶ YIELD: ABOUT 8 SERVINGS (½ CUP PER SERVING)

Protein: 4 g / Saturated Fat: < 1 g / Polyunsaturated Fat: < 1 g / Monounsaturated Fat: 1 g / Dietary Fiber: 3 g / Calories: 128

1. Put up a medium-small saucepan of water to boil, for the pasta. Preheat the oven to 350°F.

2. Heat the olive oil in a skillet with an oven-proof handle. Add the onion, and sauté over medium heat for about 5 minutes. Add the kasha or buckwheat groats, and the salt, and sauté for about 10 minutes, stirring frequently.

3. Pour in the 1¼ cups boiling water; cover and cook over low heat for about 10 minutes. Meanwhile, cook the pasta in plenty of boiling water until just tender, and drain well.

4. Stir the pasta into the kasha, cover, and bake for 30 minutes.

5. Remove from the oven, and stir in the scallions and dill. Serve hot or warm, and pass the pepper mill.

Mixed Grains with Cashews

If you want a good introduction to whole grains, this dish is it! Once cooked, the wheat becomes roly-poly and turns a beautiful warm color, and the rye puffs up and turns a lovely shade of brown. The wild rice bursts open, releasing an irresistible earthy flavor, and revealing a cream-colored interior. You can also add some barley, for extra sweetness, and, of course, the cashews provide terrific crunch. Prepare to chew! And consider using the leftovers as your whole-grain cereal for breakfast.

½ cup whole rye (also called "rye berries")

½ cup white (soft) wheat berries

¼ cup pearl barley

3½ cups water

Pinch of salt

½ cup chopped cashews, lightly toasted

- *These grains cook for the same amount of time, and therefore, can share the same pot.*

- *Make this dish in the evening and reheat it the next day. It needs a long time to cook.*

- *This dish keeps for up to 4 days stored in a tightly covered container in the refrigerator.*

▶ **YIELD: ABOUT 5 SERVINGS (¾ CUP PER SERVING)**
Protein: 8 g / Saturated Fat: 1 g / Polyunsaturated Fat: 1 g / Monounsaturated Fat: 4 g / Dietary Fiber: 7 g / Calories: 244

1. Rinse all the grains together in a strainer. Transfer to a medium-large saucepan and add 3 cups water.

2. Place the pan over medium heat and bring to a boil. Cover, then turn the heat down as far as it will go, and simmer, covered, for 1½ hours.

3. Check the grains and see if they are done to your liking. (This is a chewy pilaf.) If you would like them somewhat softer, splash in a few tablespoons of additional water, cover the pan, and continue to cook over low heat for up to 10 minutes longer. (If the grains seem about right, but there is still some water left, just turn up the heat a little, and cook them *uncovered*, stirring often, for about 5 to 10 minutes longer. The water will evaporate, but the grains will not overcook. Or you can drain out any extra water by placing the cooked grains in a colander in the sink and leaving them there for 10 minutes or so.)

4. Fluff with a fork to let steam escape, and let stand uncovered for about 10 minutes. Salt and serve hot or warm, topped with cashews.

Chocolate Meringue Cookies

These clouds of chocolate are not a dream—they are real! And you can really have them on this diet! The contrast of textures—an initial crunch, followed by a moment of chewiness—is truly satisfying, and the really good news is you can have a second one.

Nonstick spray for the baking sheet (optional)

1 cup powdered sugar

2 tablespoons unsweetened cocoa

Pinch of salt

¼ cup hazelnuts, pecans, or almonds

½ cup chocolate chips

½ teaspoon pure vanilla extract

4 egg whites (from large eggs), in a medium-large bowl

- *The baking process is slow and gradual, and the cookies keep very well in a tin or any dry, airtight container.*

- *The egg whites whip up more easily if they are at room temperature. Separate the eggs while they are still cold, placing the whites in a medium-large bowl. Cover the bowl with plastic wrap, and let it sit at room temperature for a few hours before you begin. You can discard the yolks, or find another purpose for them.*

▶ **YIELD: 1½ DOZEN (9 TWO-COOKIE SERVINGS)**

Protein: 3 g / Saturated Fat: 2 g / Polyunsaturated Fat: 1 g / Monounsaturated Fat: 2 g / Dietary Fiber: 1 g / Calories: 130

1. Preheat the oven to 250°F. Lightly spray a baking sheet with nonstick spray or line it with parchment paper.
2. Place the sugar, cocoa, salt, nuts, and chocolate chips in a food processor or blender and process in a few short bursts until the nuts and chocolate are coarsely ground.
3. Add the vanilla to the bowlful of egg whites, and beat with an electric mixer at high speed, until they form stiff peaks.
4. Pour the dry mixture on top of the beaten egg whites, and use a rubber spatula to fold everything together until reasonably well blended. (It doesn't have to be perfect.)
5. Drop by rounded tablespoons onto the prepared baking sheet.
6. Bake for 3 hours without opening the oven. Turn off the oven and leave the cookies in there for another 30 minutes. (If you forget they are there and accidentally leave them overnight, they will still be fine.) Remove the baking sheet from the oven, and let the cookies cool completely on the baking sheet before gently removing them with a metal spatula.

Coconut Macaroons

Chewy and light, these little puffs will keep for weeks if refrigerated in an airtight tin.

A little oil or melted butter for the baking sheet

3 cups shredded unsweetened coconut

1/3 cup sugar

Pinch of salt

3 large or extra-large eggs

1 teaspoon pure vanilla extract

- *You will get slightly more volume if you use extra-large eggs.*

- *This recipe can be successfully multiplied to make larger quantities*

▶ YIELD: 1½ DOZEN SMALL COOKIES
(18 ONE-COOKIE SERVINGS)

Protein: 2 g / Saturated Fat: 9.5 g / Polyunsaturated Fat: < .5 g / Monounsaturated Fat: 1 g / Dietary Fiber: 2.5 g / Calories: 131

1. Preheat the oven to 350°F. Lightly oil a baking sheet or line it with parchment paper.

2. Combine the coconut, sugar, and salt in a medium-size bowl, and mix until well combined.

3. Place the eggs and vanilla in another medium-size bowl, and beat at high speed with an electric mixer or a whisk for about 3 minutes, or until the eggs become a pale, creamy foam.

4. Add the eggs to the coconut mixture, and combine thoroughly.

5. Drop by rounded teaspoons onto the prepared baking sheet and bake on the center rack of the oven for 15 minutes, or until golden on the tops and edges.

6. Carefully remove the macaroons from the baking sheet and transfer to a wire rack. Cool completely before serving.

Honey-Broiled Pears

Sure, you could just eat a ripe pear, but sometimes you need something a little more special. Also, we all need uses for hard pears, as their perfectly ripe moment can come and go so fast, we often miss it, and then must sadly throw the fruit away.

Nonstick spray for the pan

2 medium-size firm pears

Approximately 1 tablespoon fresh lemon juice or lime juice

Approximately 1 tablespoon honey (any kind)

- *An underripe Anjou pear works very well for this, but you can use any firm variety, even Bosc.*

- *This is an opportunity to use a special honey, so if you have a gift jar left over from last holiday season, now is the time to pull it out.*

- *This dish can be made up to 2 days ahead of time and stored, tightly wrapped, in the refrigerator.*

▶ **YIELD: 2 SERVINGS**
Protein: 1 g / Saturated Fat: 0 g / Polyunsaturated Fat: 0 g / Monounsaturated Fat: 0 g / Dietary Fiber: 5 g / Calories: 130

1. Preheat the broiler to 500°F and move the oven rack to the highest position. Generously spray a glass pie pan with nonstick spray.

2. Cut the pears in half lengthwise, and remove and discard the cores. Slice each one into about six long pieces, and place them cut-side-up in the prepared pan.

3. Broil the pears for 5 to 8 minutes, depending on ripeness. (This is a very subjective process.) When the edges of the slices are tinged with a lovely golden color, and you hear sizzling, remove the pan from the broiler.

5. Push the pear slices together toward the center of the pie pan, and drizzle with about a tablespoon each of lime or lemon juice and honey. (This will be imprecise, as some of the lime juice and honey will hit the pan and sizzle. That is actually desirable.) Return the pan to the broiler.

6. After another minute or two, remove from the broiler and swish the pieces around (they will slide), and let as much of their cut surface as possible come in contact with the pan. Return to the broiler for about 2 more minutes. Watch them carefully, so the pears don't burn.

7. When the pears become exquisitely golden and crisp, they are ready to remove from the broiler. Cool in the pan, then serve warm or at room temperature.

The *Eat, Drink, and Weigh Less* Tool Kit

15

Eating Well Through Life's Ups and Downs

L IFE HAS A way of surprising you with stuff that wasn't in your plan—especially when you're on a diet. Sometimes you have to make adjustments as you go. Here's a set of tools to help:

- ► How to spot "diet food" impostors
- ► How to eat in a restaurant without blowing it
- ► How to eat on the go while managing your weight
- ► How to manage cravings

How to Spot "Diet Food" Impostors

Many foods are enthusiastically billed as "healthy" or "natural." Good though they sound, these descriptors are devoid of meaning at best and wholly misleading at worst. Become a skeptic in a good way. Don't accept clichés, assumptions, or common "wisdom." Use the information we have provided throughout this book, combined with your own common sense and powers of observation, to decide for yourself what is truly a good food choice for you.

Rule of thumb:

Be wary of "low-fat" foods (other than dairy products). Take a second look—for sugar, calories, etc.

Of course, we understand that not every crumb of every food you put in your mouth has to be an ideal nutritional specimen. There are many times when all of us just want to relax and eat something for fun. However, when we take in empty calories unconsciously and without limit, they can add up quickly and meaninglessly. Remember, when your meals and snacks are devoid of protein, healthy fat, or fiber, they will fly below your satiety radar and you'll likely eat too much and be hungry again very soon.

So we're not saying "never" with this list. We're saying, rather, open your eyes and pay attention—and don't accept clichés or hype. Be smart. That's all.

Be skeptical of:

▶ **Salads.** They are only as good for you as their actual contents. Calling something "salad" doesn't automatically mean it's a good weight-control choice. Stick mostly to leafy greens and other vegetables, and make sure the dressing isn't full of partially hydrogenated fat, sugar, refined starch, or hidden, empty calories. (See the box on page 252.)

▶ **Brown Bread.** A dark hue is not necessarily an indicator of whole-grain anything. The brown color in bread could easily be from molasses, for example. Read the nutrition panel to be sure that whole grains are indicated at or near the top of the label, in plain English. *A good rule: For every 100 calories of bread, you want to get at least 3 grams each of protein and fiber.* (See pages 264–265 for more details.)

▶ **Yogurt.** Yogurt means well. But sometimes it is so loaded with sugar that you wonder how it all fits into that little container—or how you can eat it without your teeth curling into ringlets. Read the label to make sure the yogurt is respectable. (Check out the guidelines on page 267.)

▶ **Smoothies.** Commercially prepared smoothies in little plastic bottles have become *très chic*. But beware the hidden calories in this often-faux "health food"! The protein and fiber count can be very low and the sugar count can be through the roof. Keep in mind, also, that a single container often contains two servings. (Read that label again.) In such cases, double the number of calories to get an accurate count. A better choice: homemade smoothies (pages 183–184) or plain low-fat yogurt (sweetened lightly by you, if you prefer) and a piece of whole fresh fruit, with water as your liquid. That said, there are also a (very) few decent commercially prepared smoothies on the market. (See pages 267–268 for guidelines.)

▶ **Granola.** These can vary greatly, but they all tend to be very calorie-dense. You're better off eating hot whole-grain cereals that you make yourself (pages 54–56) or a cold cereal with a good calorie-protein-fiber ratio. (See page 266.)

▶ **Muffins.** A health food hoax, for the most part. Consider them cupcakes, and (usually) very large ones at that. And unless they are labeled otherwise, you should assume that packaged muffins are loaded with trans fat. Even "low-fat" muffins are riddled with sugar and packed with calories. You're better off eating a couple of slices of whole-grain toast with low-sugar jam.

▶ **Cereal Bars and Granola Bars.** Just as muffins tend to be cupcakes with halos, cereal bars and granola bars are often indistinguishable, nutrition-wise, from cookies. Good-quality protein bars with real protein and vitamin and mineral content, less sugar, and often fewer calories, have much more to offer. We've given you some guidelines on page 268.

▶ **Fruit Juice.** This bears repeating: Fruit juice is loaded with sugar and calories—especially in the case of juice drinks. Juice is often presented as a "healthy choice," but try to avoid it, or at the very least, dilute it. The much healthier option: Eat whole fruit; drink water.

▶ **Pretzels.** A few pretzels, once in a while, can be fun to eat. But many weight-loss programs mistakenly recommend that you consider these a good snack choice on a regular basis, because they are generally fat-free or low in fat. Pretzels have nothing to offer you besides the momentary pleasure of salty, crunchy mouthfeel, and their quickly digested carbohydrates cause your blood sugar to spike (see Chapter 3). They will not only *not* fill you up, but can leave you hungrier. So, once in a while, for fun—yes, but not as a sturdy, regular solution.

▶ **Bagels.** Contrary to popular assumptions, most bagels have little or no food value and are a major empty-calorie experience. Even the dark ones are usually pretty much devoid of fiber, similar to brown bread (see opposite page). So, sorry, but these are not a good choice beyond the occasional brunch treat. On that special Sunday, you'll be better off glycemically (and sensually) if you spread your bagel lightly with cream cheese and heap on the lox, cucumbers, onions, and tomatoes.

Salad Bar Do's

Lettuce	Beans
Spinach	Tofu
Leafy greens	Cottage cheese
Raw vegetables	Hard-boiled eggs
Roasted vegetables (such as red peppers)	Sunflower seeds
	Tuna
Onions	Roasted chicken
Tomatoes	Olive oil and vinegar dressings
Lemon juice	(prepared, or make-your-own)
Edamame	

Go Easy Here

Fruit	Soy-based "bacon bits"
Hard cheeses	"Low-fat" dressings (often full of sugar)
Olives	

Salad Bar Don'ts

Sweet dressings	Crispy noodles
Bacon	Croutons
Potato salad	Other salty, crunchy doodads
Pasta salads (unless whole-grain)	

How to Eat in a Restaurant Without Blowing It

Here are some survival strategies for eating out at the most popular kinds of restaurants.

Italian/French/Continental/"Bistro"

▶ Start with a salad dressed with olive oil and vinegar (hold the croutons) or a clear, broth-based, non-creamy soup (ideally one with a few beans and lots of greens).

▶ Try to avoid the bread. If this is just too difficult and will ruin your fun (because you're the world's most passionate bread-o-phile), make a deal with yourself to "trade" the bread for rice or potatoes and/or ask the waiter not to replenish the basket after your first go-round.

▶ Ask for olive oil instead of butter.

▶ Make a choice between a pre-dinner drink and wine. Either/or—not both.

▶ Before the food arrives, have a glass of sparkling water.

▶ Instead of an entrée, order one or two appetizers or a few vegetable side dishes. Or, if you order an entrée, request an extra green vegetable instead of a starchy carbohydrate side dish.

- ▶ Split an entrée with someone else.
- ▶ Order grilled foods and ask for the sauce on the side—or better yet, just a wedge of lemon. This can be incredibly delicious!
- ▶ Eat half and take home the rest.
- ▶ Order a half portion (or child's portion) of spaghetti with red sauce, or just take three bites of someone else's pasta.
- ▶ If you can't bear the thought of skipping dessert, order one for the table and plenty of extra spoons.
- ▶ Don't forget to *eat slowly.*

Mexican/Latin

- ▶ Have a tostada instead of a burrito or enchilada–and only pretend to eat the deep-fried shell.
- ▶ ¡Beans, *sí*!
- ▶ ¡Rice, no!
- ▶ ¡Guacamole, *sí*!
- ▶ ¡Sour cream, no!
- ▶ Cheese, so-so. Keep it modest.
- ▶ Salsa is sacred (close to zero calories, tons of flavor and antioxidants), so pile it on religiously!
- ▶ If you do order a burrito, ask for it to be filled with any or all of the following: Whole beans, chicken, grilled vegetables, guacamole, and lots of salsa; but hold the rice, go light on the cheese—and throw away at least 30 percent of the flour tortilla.
- ▶ If having tacos, order the soft kind, and keep it to just two.
- ▶ One handful of chips—make them last! And ask the waiter to take the rest away or at least to the other end of the table.
- ▶ If carrying out, skip the chips. You'll get over it.

Chinese

- ▶ No white rice. Easy on the brown rice.
- ▶ No noodles.
- ▶ No deep-fried anything.
- ▶ No dough-wrapped anything.
- ▶ Try for no MSG.
- ▶ Ask them to hold the sugar. (They often will.)
- ▶ Ask for "less oil"—or ask to see the label of the oil they use and confirm it to be trans-free. You could also bring in your own healthy (peanut or canola) oil and ask them to use it! (They often will.)
- ▶ Tofu should be soft, not deep-fried.
- ▶ Eggplant can soak up a lot of calories from oil, so enjoy a small portion.

And by now, you're asking, "What's the point in eating Chinese?" Please read on:

- ▶ Soups are mostly all good. Even wonton is okay.
- ▶ Green and/or mixed vegetables with garlic are a very good choice.
- ▶ Stir-fried (unbreaded) chicken, beef, and seafood are also very good.

Japanese

- ▶ Fill up on unlimited (by anything other than your wallet) delicious miso soup and green tea!
- ▶ Avoid or minimize the rice.
- ▶ Go easy on the tempura (order an appetizer-size portion and share it).
- ▶ Order sashimi instead of sushi.
- ▶ Little appetizers (pickles, tofu, yakitori) are very good.
- ▶ Order teriyaki—ask for "light on the sauce."
- ▶ Salads tend to be very good (cold cooked spinach, seaweed, etc.). Ask for dressing—or sesame oil and vinegar—on the side.

Indian

- ▶ Skip the mango *lassi*. Order plain *lassi* or chai—and, if you need it sweet, sweeten it yourself. Otherwise, it could be supersaturated with sugar.
- ▶ Eat about a quarter of your hard-to-resist basmati rice *or* half your naan or chapati. (In other words, rice *or* bread. Not both.)
- ▶ *Pappadams* are fine in small doses.
- ▶ Deep-fried breads (such as pooris) are not fine.
- ▶ Unless you can be sure otherwise, assume that the oil in Indian restaurants is high in trans fats and avoid anything made with fat or oil, including most cooked vegetables. ("Vegetable ghee" has the highest trans-fat content we have ever measured.) If the oil is not hydrogenated, ask for less, if possible. (Some dishes are made in advance, so they're a done deal. Other times, though, they are made to order.)
- ▶ Dal and dal soup are excellent choices.
- ▶ Raita is a superb choice!
- ▶ Tandoori chicken and fish are also excellent.
- ▶ Spinach with *paneer* (a delightfully mild homemade Indian cheese) can be very good.
- ▶ Chickpea curry can be very good, too.
- ▶ Be wary of potatoes! They are often present incognito and in copious amounts.
- ▶ Be wary of eggplant! It absorbs gallons of oil.
- ▶ Skip the "deep-fried dough in syrup" dessert, rosewater or not.
- ▶ Try to eat slowly, even if there is live music. (Mollie reports that at one

of her favorite Indian restaurants in Berkeley, California, they often feature a live—and lively—sitar and tabla duo. When the music speeds up, everyone starts gulping their food really fast. So just take note, as it were.)

Thai

- ▶ Skip or minimize the rice—or ask for brown rice, which many places now offer.
- ▶ When you order Pad Thai, ask for extra tofu and vegetables.
- ▶ Coconut curries are fine. Eat them as you would a soup, to avoid needing the rice for sopping up.
- ▶ Ask for little or no sugar. Thai chefs use sugar in many recipes—and the food will taste absolutely fine without it!
- ▶ Take home the other half of your coconut-based curry (the half you didn't eat because you are so very disciplined, right?). Make this into a lovely leftover Thai dinner at home a few nights later.

Middle Eastern/Greek

- ▶ Hummus with lots of vegetables (light on the pita) is a great option.
- ▶ *Mezze* (traditional appetizer combination platter of tabouleh, hummus, tahini sauce, *tsatsiki*, and so on) can be a terrific, very satisfying shared dinner.
- ▶ Grilled chicken skewers are also very good.
- ▶ A big yes to cucumbers, tomatoes, and other salad items, especially with a tahini-based dressing.
- ▶ Load up on yogurt and yogurt sauces.
- ▶ Olive oil is fine.
- ▶ A few olives are also fine.
- ▶ If you can't resist the baklava, go ahead and order it. Ask for a very sharp knife and divide the little treasure into quarters. Share it with your dinner mates, and if you are alone, share it with the waiter (maybe leave it as part of the tip).

Coffee Bars

- ▶ Beware all yummy, frothy drinks! Go for the unsweetened options with skim milk.

Delis

- ▶ Non-creamy soups are a good choice—especially those made with lentils, barley, and/or vegetables. Consider this plus a green salad instead of an entrée.
- ▶ It's okay to have a pickle or two.
- ▶ Avoid potato salad.

- ▶ Avoid macaroni salad (unless whole-grain).
- ▶ Avoid processed meats. Go for turkey breast or lean roast beef.
- ▶ Ask for whole-grain bread, if ordering a sandwich.
- ▶ Pack any sandwich with vegetables such as romaine lettuce, spinach, onion, and cucumber, in addition to protein.
- ▶ Pack up half of your super-size sandwich and have it for dinner.
- ▶ Mustard, yes!
- ▶ Mayonnaise, modest!
- ▶ Vinegar-dressed, non-creamy coleslaw, yes—in spades!
- ▶ Creamy coleslaw in moderation.
- ▶ A few olives are fine.

Diners

- ▶ Large salads containing vegetables and maybe a few beans and a little cheese are fine. Also try a chef's salad with just the turkey and half the cheese. Dress with oil and vinegar—or, if using a commercial dressing, go lightly, or ask for it on the side.
- ▶ Breakfast at odd hours can be fun. Poached eggs or lightly scrambled eggs with whole-grain toast (hold the potatoes!) at 2:00 P.M. or 8:00 P.M. are terrific with a generous mound of salsa.
- ▶ Go for a side of cottage cheese.
- ▶ Cooked green vegetables with olive oil are fine.
- ▶ Grilled chicken or fish are good choices. No breading, though.
- ▶ If you feel the need to order a baked potato, share it with one or two other people. Try seasoning it with olive oil, salsa, or black pepper instead of sour cream. Or, if you use sour cream, ask for it on the side, and dab—rather than dump—it on.
- ▶ Avoid the rolls—chances are they will be very white and nutrient-empty.

Fast Food—If You Must . . .

. . . But only when starvation is the alternative. We have indicated the least-bad choices, all of which will keep you at around 400 calories or less.

Most of the fast-food chains are now offering salads. Having them with grilled chicken may not be the greatest culinary experience, but it can be an okay meal. Do include some salad dressing (as long as it's not full of partially hydrogenated fat, sugar, or refined starch) and avoid the croutons. It's fine to consider this a full meal (checking the calorie count, if you wish, to see how it fits into your daily plan). Please note that skipping the salad dressing and going for very low calories is not a great strategy, as this will leave you hungry before too long.

- Plain burger with half or none of the bun (condiments okay)
- Grilled or broiled chicken (ditto on the bun and condiments)
- "Veggie" burgers (ditto on the bun and condiments)—if edible
- Salads (minus the croutons and with a nonsweet dressing)
- Scrambled eggs
- "Pita" offerings (as in Jack in the Box's Chicken Fajita Pita or Southwest Pita)
- Thin-crusted plain pizza (as in 2 slices of Domino's Crunchy Thin Crust or 1 slice Pizza Hut's Thin & Crispy "Veggie Lovers")
- Subway—Veggie Delight; Deli Ham; Deli Turkey Breast. Sandwiches can be whole-grain and tailored, including hollowing out the bread, adding more vegetables, and using less mayonnaise.
- Taco Bell—Fresco Style menu

Eating on the Go While Managing Your Weight

Knowing how, what, and where to eat decently while you are out and about can be one of the best tools for maintaining the wonderfully trimmed and toned body you are acquiring through the 21-Day Diet and our other eating plans. Weight management and healthy eating are as portable as you are organized and willing. Invest in some good food-packing supplies and decide that you really don't mind being known as that rather odd person who is always carrying around her own food. Who knows? Maybe you'll become known as a trend-setter and plastic food containers will soon become as fashionable as designer water bottles. Besides, they'll make a smashing accessory to your own great new look, as you slim down and glow with shining health. (For menus, see the Portable Plan, pages 134–140.)

Discover "Deliberate Leftovers"

Now that you're becoming a well-versed healthy menu-planner and cook, get into the habit of making more food than you can eat at one meal. We call this creating deliberate leftovers, and they're the best way to keep yourself eating well and affordably no matter where you are. Anticipate the days when you'll be away from your kitchen or cafeteria at mealtime, and pack up the extra food for these times.

The Road Plan

For those of you who spend a lot of time driving, don't fill up at the "snack mart" where you stop to fill up the car. Instead, here are some things you can do to keep your eating healthy and on track.

▶ *May the cooler be with you.* If you are a car commuter, it can make a very big (and positive) difference to adopt a small cooler for toting real food—your deliberate leftovers or a Very Tall Sandwich (page 155), for example—and high-quality one-handed snacks (fresh fruit, baby carrots, small pull-top cans of tomato juice, and so on). Make it part of your routine to refreeze your plastic ice pack each night just as regularly as you charge your cell phone. This is also a good plan for an errand day, carpooling, or just general traipsing around.

▶ *Make that road trip into a picnic.* For long road trips, consider packing a basket of delights. This takes a bit of advance planning, shopping, and preparing, but it can be a truly enjoyable ritual—and a very economical and refreshing departure from truck stops and other unpredictable, not to mention unpoetic, places to stop and grab possibly inedible fare.

The Air Plan

Even when airlines used to serve real meals, it was by and large a sad story. Nevertheless, those of us who brown-bagged it on the plane were looked at askance by our aisle mates. (In all fairness, it could have been the fumes from the dill pickles. But still.) Nowadays, it is much more common to carry one's own food on planes, as there is often no other option beyond the sad little snack boxes they offer—or have the nerve to charge you for. Still, be wary of the packaged foods sold at airports (very cleverly, in many cases, right at the gate) or in the plane itself. These tend to be ridiculously expensive and caloric—and will rarely have good nutritional content. It's always better to plan, prepare, and pack your own. A carry-on bag filled with food is a great idea and it's really worth the trouble. Here are some suggestions:

▶ *Breakfast on the fly.* For a morning flight, pack some high-quality whole-grain cereal in a plastic container with a tight-fitting lid. When the beverage cart arrives, ask for some milk (it's all low-fat these days) and just pour it into your container. Voilà! Breakfast! (Don't forget to carry a plastic spoon.)

▶ *Pack your bags, then pack a sandwich.* Make yourself a sandwich on whole-grain bread, packing some of the more perishable or delicate components separately (i.e., put the lettuce, tomato, and other vegetables in a sealed plastic bag, so they will stay crisp. Wrap each half of the sandwich separately and tightly in plastic wrap, or pack the sandwich in a sandwich-shaped hard-plastic container with a tight-fitting lid to keep it from getting crushed).

▶ *Take back the snack.* Carry a nice little chunk of good cheese (it stays good for a day at room temperature), some Super Trail Mix (page 176) in a sealed plastic bag, a couple of apples, assorted cut vegetables in another sealed plastic bag, and whole-grain crackers—and don't forget a nice piece or two of dark chocolate. Also, a good-quality protein bar (page 268) can be a very decent "meal solution" for travelers. This way, you are not only going to eat better, but you will be on your own schedule—not at the mercy of whether they might or might not happen to be coming around with their dubious snacks.

▶ *Get the best of the beverage cart.* Drinks that are food: Tomato juice. Milk. That's about it. (And to make this even more limiting, be aware that tomato juice is usually extremely high in sodium, so you don't want to be chugging it down in large quantities.) These are your best choices, in addition to bottled water (which is really the best choice, especially when accented with a wedge of lemon or lime). Easy on the orange juice and other fruit juices. Remember, they're full of sugar, so if you crave them, consider diluting them greatly with sparkling water. They're much more thirst-quenching that way.

The Workplace Plan

▶ *Bring your lunch.* This requires some planning. We're here to help! (See pages 155–174 for ideas.) Besides saving you lots of money, packing a lunch lets you be in complete control of portion size and nutritional content.

▶ *Make the most of the kitchenette.* If you're lucky, your workplace will have a refrigerator and a microwave. Make both a part of your routine so you can enjoy a nice, warm, sustaining lunch (especially one that relies on deliberate leftovers).

▶ *Lunch meeting strategy.* Go for non-creamed soups, salad with oil and vinegar dressing, fruit salad, and sandwiches made with whole-grain bread, if possible. Try to eat just half a sandwich, and go back for seconds on fruit salad. When they bring out the cookies, eat just half of one.

The Straight-Out-of-the-Supermarket Plan

Okay, so you're just not a born food carrier. Not everyone is. Don't feel discouraged if you are not inclined to do all the planning, preparing, and packing described above. Here's another alternative: Stop and buy your on-the-go foods at supermarkets. This will often be a much more affordable and healthful solution than getting your lunch at restaurants or cafés on the fly. Our recommendations:

- *Drop in at the deli.* Order the closest approximation they have to a Very Tall Sandwich (page 155). (You can ask them to stuff it with many extra vegetables.) Or try some plain, sliced deli meat or some roasted chicken.
- *Belly up to the salad bar.* Buy a small container of cut-up vegetables or fruit salad as a snack or light meal. Salads that you fix yourself are ideal, or you can buy a prepared one that looks fresh and isn't smothered with a creamy dressing or sauce. If you are a vegetarian, be sure to include some beans, nuts, and/or hard-boiled eggs. A touch of cheese is also fine.
- *Pick produce.* Stop by the produce section and stock up on baby carrots and other cut vegetables (increasingly available). Choose some fresh fruit (whole, such as apples, peaches, cherries, or berries; or cut-up fruit, such as melon halves, which you can eat with a spoon).
- *Dairy to be different.* The dairy aisle offers high-protein quick fixes, such as low-fat milk, decent yogurts (see page 267), and small containers of cottage cheese. Mozzarella sticks can also be handy.
- *Grab and go natural.* If you are in a big "grab and go" hurry, do your grabbing at the natural foods fridge. Reach for a neat little rectangular shrink-wrap of baked tofu (quite tasty straight from the package) or a container of hummus or bean dip. Grab some fresh salsa while you're at it, too.
- *Say yes to a snack bar.* While you're running to the check-out counter, you can also grab a respectable protein bar. Just make sure it's one that really delivers, nutritionally speaking (see page 268).

The Convenience Store Survival Guide
(Last, and Definitely Least, but Better than Something Worse)

- Apples
- Oranges
- Bananas
- Packaged nuts
- Packaged trail mix (look for those with more nuts and fewer raisins and sugared fruit)
- Peanuts in shell
- Sunflower seeds in shell
- Pistachios in shell
- "Good" chips—many chips are now trans fat–free, and make a decent snack if limited to small (1- to 2-ounce) servings. SunChips deserve a special note, as they are whole-grain and made with healthy fats.
- Good-quality protein bars (see page 268)
- Good-quality yogurt (see page 267)

- ▶ Good-quality smoothies (see pages 267–268)
- ▶ A carton of low-fat or skim milk
- ▶ A loaf of whole-grain bread with a good profile (see pages 264–265)—eat some now, and take the rest home.
- ▶ A small jar of peanut butter (and a plastic knife), to go along with the bread
- ▶ Packaged cut vegetables
- ▶ Special K in an eat-in-the-pack arrangement (better calorie and protein counts than instant oatmeal), while not terrific, is always there for you if you are desperate. Eat with low-fat or skim milk.
- ▶ Fresh sandwiches and wraps

If you have access to a microwave:

- ▶ A small can of chili
- ▶ Just-add-water, eat-in-the-pack soups. Avoid noodle soups, which tend to have no nutritional value and loads of sodium, and opt for split pea, lentil, or anything with beans.
- ▶ A can of soup. Go for bean or lentil. Avoid "cream of anything" or anything with noodles.
- ▶ Quaker Oatmeal Express. Eat with low-fat or skim milk.

How to Manage Cravings

It can be sudden and overwhelming—that seemingly irresistible desire to tear into a bag of corn chips or inhale a whole box of Ho Hos. Just as when we meditate, we can become neutral, nonjudging observers of our less-than-lofty thoughts as they come and go, we also have it within ourselves to stand outside our extracurricular food urges until they subside. And they usually do subside.

This brings to mind the "three-minute mantra" often invoked in smoking cessation workshops, which goes something like: "A nicotine craving lasts for three minutes. So it's not about how to get through *life* without cigarettes, it's more about getting through the next *three minutes* without *this* cigarette."

Yes, the good news is, cravings dissipate. The not-so-good news is that they also return. It's just one of those plain facts of life. But the *ultimate* good news is that there are tools we can acquire that will not only help us avert a meltdown, but even allow us to keep a sense of humor about it all—and stay on track.

- ▶ *Give yourself a time-out.* Take a few deep breaths and pour yourself a glass of cold water. Better yet, make yourself a cup of herbal tea. (Licorice tea mixed with a little peppermint can be very perky—and is naturally sweet.) Try to figure out if you are really hungry or just bored or lonely. All too often, if you are eating from an emotional cue, the more you eat, the worse you feel. Try writing down your feelings—or a list of things you'd like to do, or even a shopping list of groceries or craft supplies, or fun home improvement, gardening, or office items. Scotch tape is a nice diversion. So are colored paper clips. Or how about a really good book or a CD of samba music? You get the drift.

▶ **Bag a bad habit.** Becoming conscious of a negative eating pattern is the first step to getting on top of it—and once you do, you'll realize that what felt like a craving was just a habit. One of Mollie's friends, a stay-at-home mom who is with her children (and their favorite crummy snack foods) during the afterschool and early evening hours each day puts it this way: "I couldn't resist those big bags of junk cookies where you get, like, four hundred of them for three dollars. But, you know, I decided that avoiding this didn't require some big mystical insight. I mean, what I needed to do was just not open my mouth. Period." So she did. Not open her mouth, that is. She just cold-turkeyed the habit. And she reported that by as early as day two, it was no longer an issue.

GO FOR THE FORK IN THE ROAD INSTEAD OF THE FORK

FOUR OR FIVE times a week Katherine will eat ice cream late at night (a third of a pint at a time). She does not particularly enjoy it. After keeping a food journal for just a few days and trying the Warm-Up Plan for a week, she figured out how to take control of this craving.

"Find things that you like to do—things that engage your mind and don't include food," she recommends. For Katherine, this means playing the guitar or drawing. When she feels the ice cream urge coming on, she'll take the Ben & Jerry's out of the freezer and set it on the counter to begin softening. Then she'll go play the guitar or draw for a while, and will experience a feeling of satisfaction. More often than not, she says, the desire for the ice cream will fade and she'll end up putting it back into the freezer unopened. Lately, she has stopped buying the ice cream altogether and finds that she doesn't miss it.

Katherine's advice: Turn off the TV and do something more mentally involving. If necessary, make a list of things you like to do and refer to your list if you have a blank moment. This has helped Katherine go from choosing a zoned-out state of eating and TV to choosing a zoned-in state of activity.

▶ **Cook away cravings.** It might seem odd, if not downright counter-intuitive, but cooking can actually avert an eating binge. Take out your pots and pans and dive into a whole new relationship with food. It can be a remarkably effective way to become more conscious about food by applying a different, more creative part of your brain to it. You don't just reach for it, you *participate* in it—and thus appreciate it more.

▶ *Snack mindfully.* Pour a glass of water first, then prepare yourself a lovely platter of, say, baby carrots, with a scattering of raisins and a few almonds. Don't eat it yet! Sit down, take a deep breath, and drink all the water first. Take a few more breaths, then eat the carrots and raisins and almonds slowly, one by one. Drink more water. Sit and breathe a little more.

▶ *Brush your teeth.* Seriously! It's a very effective strategy for riding out a craving.

▶ *Revisit your diet.* Maybe, when you experience cravings, it is for the simple, straightforward reason that you are not eating enough nutritious food. Daily caloric needs are a very personal thing. There is no "one size fits all" template. And such needs can wax and wane, depending on activity, stress level, and other factors. If you are currently following the 21-Day Diet, remember that it is quite low in calories, and perhaps you need a bit more. Try beefing up your protein intake (so to speak) or drizzling a little more olive oil onto your delicious green vegetable. Have more of the vegetable itself, while you're at it. Add another serving of fresh fruit with some good yogurt to your daily snack. You can deliciously augment your healthy intake without adding empty calories. And the more you satisfy your nutritional needs, the less you'll reach for nutrition-challenged food-shaped objects when you feel yourself flagging.

▶ *Sometimes you really want what you think you want.* All of the above notwithstanding, sometimes you just want that chocolate, period. It's not about existential longing or latent frustration—it's truly about the Hershey's Kiss. Well, have it! Have several. But let yourself enjoy the experience. Eat slowly and deliberately—and really *taste* the chocolate. And if you need a safety net under your eating urges, see page 109 for some simple guidelines to allow "That Thing You Crave" into the diet itself without causing the sky to fall.

16

Shopping Guide

TIPS ON SELECTING SOME OF THE MORE CONFUSING ITEMS

BRING YOUR GLASSES to the store when shopping for breads, cereals, crackers, bars, yogurt, smoothies, and "veggie burgers." The calorie counts and nutritional profiles of these items can vary wildly. In this handy list, we've done a lot of the legwork for you, pointing out the most important features and brands to look for. Don't bother counting total fat, carbohydrates, or sugar grams (except when indicated otherwise, as with yogurt and smoothies). Just check these numbers and remember also to double-check the size of a serving. Some labeling can be deceptive.

Sliced Bread

What to look for:
- ▶ Whole grains at the top of the ingredients list
- ▶ 90–110 calories per slice (or less, if you can find it)
- ▶ 3 or more grams of protein per slice
- ▶ 3 or more grams of fiber per slice

Examples:

- *Rudi's Organic Bakery*
  Right Choice series and Whole Grains & Fiber series
- *Country Hearth*
  Stone Ground 100% Whole Wheat
- *Sara Lee*
  Heart Healthy Multi-Grain
  Heart Healthy Homestyle 100% Whole Wheat
- *Earthgrains*
  Extra Fiber 100% Whole Wheat
  Extra Fiber 100% Multi-Grain
- *Pepperidge Farm*
  100% Whole Wheat Thin Sliced
  Carb-Style Soft 100% Whole Wheat
  7 Grain Lifeworks Wheat or Seven Grain
  Natural Whole Grain series
  Very Thin Sliced Whole Wheat

English Muffins

What to look for:
- ▶ Whole grains at the top of the ingredients list
- ▶ 130 or fewer calories per muffin
- ▶ 4 or more grams of protein
- ▶ 3 or more grams of fiber

Examples:
- Thomas' Hearty Grain 100% Whole Wheat
- Thomas' Hearty Grain 12 Grain

Burger Buns

What to look for:
- ▶ Whole grains at the top of the ingredients list
- ▶ 110 or fewer calories per bun
- ▶ 3 or more grams of protein per bun
- ▶ 3 or more grams of fiber per bun

Examples:
- Roman Meal Multi-Grain Hamburger Buns
- Rudi's Organic Bakery "Right Choice" Hamburger Buns

Breakfast Cereals

What to look for:
- ▶ Whole grains at the top of the ingredients list
- ▶ 150 or fewer calories per serving. (Check the box to know the volume of 1 serving. Sometimes it's only ½ cup.)
- ▶ 4 or more grams of protein per serving
- ▶ 3 or more grams of fiber per serving

Examples:
Cold cereal
- All-Bran Original
- Wheaties
- Whole Grain Total
- Kashi GOLEAN
- Barbara's Multigrain Shredded Spoonfuls

Hot cereal
- Wheatena
- Bob's Red Mill 7-Grain
- Kashi Breakfast Pilaf
- McCann's Original Steel-Cut Irish Oatmeal
- Old-Fashioned Quaker Oats
- Kashi Heart to Heart Instant Oatmeal
  Or cook your own whole grains (see pages 54–56). It's cheaper, more varied—and just plain better!

Whole-Grain Crackers

What to look for:
- ▶ Whole grains at the top of the ingredients list
- ▶ 130 or fewer calories per serving. (Check the box to know the volume of 1 serving.)
- ▶ No trans fats

Examples:
- Kashi TLC, any flavor
- Ak-Mak 100% Whole Wheat Stone Ground Sesame Crackers
- Trader Joe's Semi-Precious Mini Stone Wheat Crackers
- Wheat Thins Multi-Grain
- Triscuit Thin Crisps

Yogurt

What to look for per 6-ounce serving:
- ▶ 100 or fewer calories
- ▶ 14 or fewer grams of sugar
- ▶ 5 or more grams of protein

Keep in mind that, unless otherwise specified, most flavored nonfat or low-fat yogurt is loaded with sugar and quite high in calories! The ideal way to control the calories in yogurt is to purchase a good brand of low-fat or nonfat plain. If you like it sweet, then you can sweeten (and flavor) it yourself with fruit, or a little honey or sugar—or a small amount of non-caloric sweetener. If that is just too inconvenient and you need to find something sweet directly from the supermarket shelf, look for the brands that are sweetened with less sugar.

Examples:
- Total 0%
- Dannon*
  - Light 'n Fit Carb Control (all flavors)
  - Light 'n Fit (all flavors)
  - Light 'n Fit Creamy (all flavors)
- Stonyfield Farm "MOOve Over Sugar" (all flavors)
- Yoplait Light* (all flavors)

Smoothies

The first and best option is to make your own (pages 182–184). But if you need to grab one from the grocery store, keep in mind that many commercially prepared "healthy" drinks are deceptively packaged (the nutrition panel will often give numbers for only half the contents) and tend to be high in sugar and calories.

What to look for per 10-ounce bottle:
- ▶ 130 or fewer calories
- ▶ 9 or more grams of protein
- ▶ 19 or fewer grams of sugar

Examples:
Stonyfield Farm Light Smoothie† (all flavors)

---

*Note that other versions of Dannon and Yoplait contain a great deal of sugar, so be sure to look for "Light 'n Fit" (Dannon) or "Light" (Yoplait) on the label.

†Make sure it's "Light" and not "Lowfat," which is a different product and contains more calories and sugar.

Yoplait Smoothie Light (all flavors)
Dannon Light 'n Fit Smoothie (all flavors)

Good-Quality Protein Bars

Many—even most—"energy bars" are not nutritious at all. But some are actually good for you and can deliver a respectable dose of protein, vitamins, and minerals without too much sugar thrown in on the sly.

What to look for per bar:
- ▶ 200 or fewer calories
- ▶ 10 or more grams of protein
- ▶ 10 or fewer grams of sugar
- ▶ 2 or more grams of fiber
- ▶ No trans fat

Examples:
- • Pria Complete Nutrition Bar (all flavors)
- • Pria CarbSELECT (all flavors)
- • LUNA (all flavors)
- • Kashi GOLEAN Crunchy Bar
- • Kashi GOLEAN Rolls

Burgers

In the 21-Day Diet, "burger," can mean meat (lean ground turkey or 90 to 95% lean beef) or "veggie." Vegetable burger options are all over the map these days, so here are some helpful guidelines:

What to look for:
- ▶ 100 or fewer calories (Bonus: If they're 80 or under, you can have two.)
- ▶ 11 or more grams of protein

Examples:
- • BOCA Burgers
    All-American Meatless Flame Grilled
    Boca Original
    Grilled Vegetable
    Roasted Onion
    Roasted Garlic
- • Morningstar Farms
    Better'n Burgers

- Gardenburger
    Original
    Sun-Dried Tomato-Basil
    Veggie Medley
    Black Bean
- Natural Touch Vegan Burger
- Note:
    For vegetarian "ground beef," try BOCA Meatless Ground Burger or Morningstar Farms Grillers Burger Style or Sausage Style Recipe Crumbles.

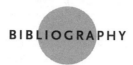

BIBLIOGRAPHY

Albert, C. M., et al. "Blood Levels of Long-Chain n-3 Fatty Acids and the Risk of Sudden Death." *New England Journal of Medicine* 346 (2002):1113–18.

Appel, L. J., et al. "A Clinical Trial of the Effects of Dietary Patterns on Blood Pressure." *New England Journal of Medicine* 336 (1997):1117–24.

Bischoff-Ferrari, H. A., et al. "Positive Association Between 245-Hydroxy Vitamin D Levels and Bone Mineral Density: A Population-Based Study of Younger and Older Adults." *American Journal of Medicine* 116 (2004):634–39.

Botto, L. D., et al. "Neural-Tube Defects." *New England Journal of Medicine* 341 (1999):1509–19.

Brown, L., et al. "A Prospective Study of Carotenoid Intake and Risk of Cataract Extraction in U.S. Men." *American Journal of Clinical Nutrition* 70 (1999):517–24.

Calle, E. E., et al. "Overweight, Obesity, and Mortality from Cancer in a Prospectively Studied Cohort of U.S. Adults." *New England Journal of Medicine* 348 (2003):1625–38.

Chan, J. M., et al. "Dairy Products, Calcium, and Prostate Cancer Risk in the Physicians' Health Study." *American Journal of Clinical Nutrition* 74 (2001):549–54.

Cho, E., et al. "Dairy Foods, Calcium, and Colorectal Cancer: A Pooled Analysis of 10 Cohort Studies." *Journal of the National Cancer Institute* 96 (2004):1015–22.

Curhan, G. C., et al. "Prospective Study of Beverage Use and the Risk of Kidney Stones." *American Journal of Epidemiology* 143 (1999):240–47.

Dietary Guidelines for Americans 2005. Washington, D.C.: U.S. Department of Agriculture. 2005. http://www.healthierus.gov/dietaryguidelines

Drewnowski, A. "Obesity and the Food Environment: Dietary Energy Density and Diet Costs." *American Journal of Preventive Medicine* 27 (2004):154–62.

Feskanich, D., et al. "Calcium, Vitamin D, Milk Consumption, and Hip Fractures: A Prospective Study Among Postmenopausal Women." *American Journal of Clinical Nutrition* 77 (2003):504–11.

Feskanich, D., et al. "Plasma Vitamin D Metabolites and Risk of Colorectal Cancer in Women." *Cancer Epidemiology, Biomarkers and Prevention* 13 (2004):1502–8.

Feskanich, D., et al. "Walking and Leisure-Time Activity and Risk of Hip Fracture in Post-menopausal Women." *Journal of the American Medical Association* 288 (2002):2300–6.

Fung, T. T., et al. "Dietary Patterns, Meat Intake, and the Risk of Type 2 Diabetes in Women." *Archives of Internal Medicine* 164 (2004):2235–40.

Giovannucci, E. "Tomatoes, Tomato-Based Products, Lycopene, and Cancer: Review of the Epidemiologic Literature." *Journal of the National Cancer Institute* 91 (1999):317–31.

Grodstein, F., et al. "A Large Randomized Trial of Beta-Carotene Supplements and Cognitive Function." *Neurobiology of Aging* 25 (suppl 2) (2004):54.

Hedley, A. A., et al. "Prevalence of Overweight and Obesity Among U.S. Children, Adolescents, and Adults, 1999-2002." *Journal of the American Medical Association* 291 (2004):2847–50.

Hercberg, S., et al. "The SU.VI.MAX Study: A Randomized, Placebo-Controlled Trial of the Health Effects of Antioxidant Vitamins and Minerals." *Archives of Internal Medicine* 164 (2004):2335–42.

Holmes, M. D., et al. "Association of Dietary Intake of Fat and Fatty Acids with Risk of Breast Cancer." *Journal of the American Medical Association* 281 (1999):914–20.

Hu, F. B. "Plant-Based Foods and Prevention of Cardiovascular Disease: An Overview." *American Journal of Clinical Nutrition* 78 (suppl) (2003):544–51.

Hu, F. B., et al. "Dietary Fat Intake and the Risk of Coronary Heart Disease in Women." *New England Journal of Medicine* 337 (1997):1491–99.

Hu, F. B., et al. "Frequent Nut Consumption and Risk of Coronary Heart Disease in Women: Prospective Cohort Study." *British Medical Journal* 317 (7169) (1998): 1341–45.

Hu, F. B., et al. "A Prospective Study of Egg Consumption and Risk of Cardiovascular Disease in Men and Women." *Journal of the American Medical Association* 281 (1999):1387–94.

Liu, S., et al. "A Prospective Study of Dietary Glycemic Load, Carbohydrate Intake and Risk of Coronary Heart Disease in U.S. Women." *American Journal of Clinical Nutrition* 71 (2000):1455–61.

McCullough, M. L., et al. "Diet Quality and Major Chronic Disease Risk in Men and Women: Moving Toward Improved Dietary Guidance." *American Journal of Clinical Nutrition* 76 (2002):1261–71.

Mukamel, K. J., et al. "Roles of Drinking Pattern and Type of Alcohol Consumed in Coronary Heart Disease in Men." *New England Journal of Medicine* 348 (2003):109–18.

Trichopoulou, A., et al. "Adherence to a Mediterranean Diet and Survival in a Greek Population." *New England Journal of Medicine* 348 (2003):2599–608.

White, L. R., et al. "Brain Aging and Midlife Tofu Consumption." *Journal of the American College of Nutrition* 19 (2000):242–55.

Willett, W. *Nutritional Epidemiology*, second edition. New York: Oxford University Press, 1998.

Willett, W. C., et al. "Guidelines for Healthy Weight." *New England Journal of Medicine* 341 (1999): 427–34.

Yamamoto, S., et al. "Soy, Isoflavones, and Breast Cancer Risk in Japan." *Journal of the National Cancer Institute* 95 (2003):906–13.

Zhang, S., et al. "A Prospective Study of Folate Intake and the Risk of Breast Cancer." *Journal of the American Medical Association* 281 (1999):1632–37.

INDEX

fruit(s), 7, 14, 19–33, 36, 49, 52, 91
  A-list, 30
  B-list, 30
  colors of, 28
  dried, 31
  in *Eat, Drink, and Weigh Less* Pyramid, 14
  exotic, black beans with, 162
  families of, 25–26
  frozen, 28, 29
  increasing intake of, 32
  nutrients in, 22–23, 28
  preparation of, 21
  servings of, 32
fruit drinks, 69, 91, 251
fruit juice, 31, 67–68, 69, 71, 72, 74, 91, 251

galactose, 51
gallstones, 9, 70, 75
garbanzo beans (chickpeas), 59, 62
  easy three-bean chili, 211
  hummus, 190
garlic
  roasted, paste, 185
  roasted, vinaigrette, 198
gas, 27–28
gazpacho, 174
glucose (dextrose), 11, 49, 50, 51, 52, 71
glycemic index and glycemic load, 50–51, 52
glycogen, 11, 49
grain dishes
  bulgur-pine nut pilaf, 240
  bulgur with olive oil and lemon, 239
  kasha varnishkes, 242
  millet and quinoa with toasted sunflower
    seeds, 241
  mixed grains with cashews, 243
  whole-wheat couscous with pistachios and
    orange zest, 238
grains, 49
  protein in, 59
  refined, 51, 52
grains, whole, 7, 15, 36, 49, 50, 52–57, 64, 91
  buying, 53
  cooking, 53, 54–56
  crackers, 266
  in *Eat, Drink, and Weigh Less* Pyramid, 14
  food packages and, 56
  see also bread, whole-grain; grain dishes;
    specific grains
granola, 250–51
granola bars, 251
grapefruit juice, 71
gravy, amazing, 196
  mushroom, 197
Greek restaurants, 255
green beans
  in crunchy peanut coating with protein-of-

  choice, 218–19
  five-minute flash-cooked, 234
  Thai-inspired red curry, 222
greens
  braised, with walnuts and sour cherries, 231
  buckwheat noodles with cashews and, 216

hamburger, 60
Health Professionals' Follow-up Study, xii, 29,
  71, 85
"healthy food" imposters, 249–51
healthy weight, 8–9, 15
heart disease (cardiovascular disease), xii, 3, 9,
  10, 15, 19, 22, 29, 52
  alcohol and, 75, 76, 77
  carbohydrates and, 50
  eggs and, 46
  fats and, 35, 36, 40, 41, 42, 43
  French paradox and, 75
  Mediterranean diet and, 37
  n-3 fats and, 45–46
  nuts and seeds and, 62
  physical activity and, 83, 85
  salt and, 72
  sodas and, 68
  vitamin E and, 80
heart rhythm, 23, 36, 45
high-fructose corn syrup, 69
honey
  -broiled pears, 246
  mustard dressing, 200
honeydew smoothie, 183
hummus, 190
hunger, 88–90, 91–92
  thirst and, 67, 90, 92
hydration, 15, 66–74, 89

ice cream, 52
Indian restaurants, 254–55
insulin, 26, 40, 49, 50, 52, 68, 86, 89
  snacks and, 93
Italian restaurants, 252–53
Italian-style pan-sautéed broccoli, 232

Japanese restaurants, 254
juices
  fruit, 31, 67–68, 69, 71, 72, 74, 91, 251
  vegetable, 69

kamut, 56
kasha (buckwheat groats), 54, 55, 62
  varnishkes, 242
kidney stones, 70, 71
knives, 21

Latin restaurants, 253
leftovers, 257